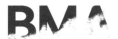

The Practical Pocket Guide to History Taking and Clinical Examination

TIMOTHY WILLIAMSON

MBChB, BSc (Hons)

NIHR Academic Clinical Fellow in Medical Education
University of Leicester, UK

and

LESLEY THOMS

BSc (Hons)

Final Year Medical Student
University of Leicester, UK

D1380444

Radcliffe Publishing
London • New York

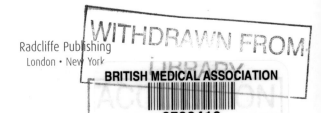

Radcliffe Publishing Ltd
St Mark's House
Shepherdess Walk
London N1 7BQ
United Kingdom

www.radcliffehealth.com

British Library Cataloguing in Publication Data

A catalogue record for this book is available from the British Library.

ISBN-13: 978 190891 155 1

The paper used for the text pages of this book is FSC® certified. FSC (The Forest Stewardship Council®) is an international network to promote responsible management of the world's forests.

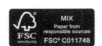

Typeset by Beautiful Words, Auckland, New Zealand
Manufacturing managed by 21six

Contents

Preface

There are many books in circulation that provide detailed explanations of clinical history taking and examination. This book serves as a reference tool for trainees of various disciplines to refine their skills in this area. By listing the questions required for a focused history, as well as the key components of the ideal examination, readers can develop clinical skills that are both relevant and succinct.

To ensure a detailed and specific history, this book has been reviewed by 31 practising clinicians of various specialties, nationwide. Their contributions have been pivotal in developing this concise yet comprehensive pocketbook for training and clinical practice.

The Practical Pocket Guide to History Taking and Clinical Examination aims to:

➲ guide the reader to develop concise and detailed history and examination skills

➲ function as an aide memoire for clinical practice and exam preparation

➲ serve as a tool to cross-reference histories and examinations performed.

Timothy Williamson
Lesley Thoms
May 2014

About the authors

Dr Timothy Williamson worked for six years as a Royal Naval Medic and graduated in Pharmacology from the University of Bath (2004), before completing his MBChB at the University of Warwick (2009). He won various scholarships and awards at medical school, including the Pridgeon Gold Medal for Research. After graduation his positions have focused on medical education. He has held an academic foundation post as a Clinical Educator, followed by an Academic Clinical Fellowship in Medical Education in the Department of Medical and Social Care Education at the University of Leicester.

Lesley Thoms is currently a final year medical student on the graduate entry programme at the University of Leicester. She has a first class honours degree in Psychology and has worked in the field prior to studying medicine. Lesley has many years' experience within the mental health sector and within social scientific research, working to promote patient experience and quality healthcare. Lesley will soon start an academic foundation position in Leadership and Management at the University Hospitals of Leicester NHS Trust.

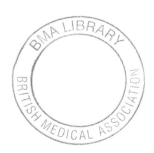

List of contributors

Christopher Aitchison
Paramedic Lecturer
Scottish Ambulance Academy

Jonathan Barratt
Honorary Consultant Nephrologist
Leicester General Hospital, UK

Rachael Boddy
Consultant in Emergency Medicine
Heartlands Hospital, UK

Anna Carter
Graduate Entry Medical Student
University of Nottingham, UK

Roger Cooke
Consultant in Occupational
Medicine
Worcester, UK

Sarah Cross
Senior Lecturer in Emergency,
Paramedical and Urgent Care
University of Northampton, UK

Michael Ferguson
Consultant in Anaesthetics & ITU
Leicester Royal Infirmary, UK

Savio Fernandes
Consultant in Haematology
Dudley Group Foundation NHS Trust,
UK

David Fitzpatrick
Paramedic Clinical Research
Specialist
University of Stirling, UK

Beth Goundry
Core Medical Trainee
West Sussex Healthcare Trust, UK

Robert Haughney
Consultant in Obstetrics and
Gynaecology
Kettering Hospital, UK

Neil Johnson
General Practitioner
Warwickshire, UK

Ashley Knights
Paramedic Lecturer
University of Northampton, UK

Arlena Kuenzel
Foundation Doctor
Belfast University Hospitals, UK

Matthew Lawrence
Acute Care Common Stem
Trainee
Glasgow Hospitals, UK

Nick London
Professor of Vascular Surgery
University of Leicester, UK

Robert Maher
Graduate Entry Medical
Student
University of Nottingham, UK

David Metcalfe
Academic Clinical Fellow in Trauma
& Orthopaedic Surgery
University of Warwick, UK

Andrew Miller
Consultant Lower Gastrointestinal
Surgeon
University Hospitals of Leicester,
UK

Jonathan Murray
Specialist Registrar in Psychiatry
Leicestershire Primary Care Trust,
UK

Khrystle Nazaire
Foundation Doctor
London, UK

Katherine Nichol
Specialist Registrar in General
Practice
Queen Elizabeth Hospital NHS Trust,
King's Lynn, UK

Sophie O'Dowd
Specialist Registrar in Radiology
Royal Derby Hospitals, UK

Henry Pau
Professor of ENT Surgery
University Hospitals of Leicester,
UK

Colin Read
Consultant in Emergency Medicine
Morecambe Bay NHS Foundation
Trust, UK

Frances Rees
Specialist Registrar in Rheumatology
Queen's Medical Centre,
Nottingham, UK

John Rogers
Core Medical Trainee
Bristol Hospitals, UK

Marion Sikuade
Specialist Registrar in
Ophthalmology
Royal Hallamshire Hospital,
Sheffield, UK

Paul Sooby
Core Surgical Trainee
East Sussex NHS Healthcare Trust,
UK

Clare Sutton
Paramedic Practice Educator
University of Northampton, UK

Patrick Wheeler
Consultant and Senior Clinical
Fellow in Sport and Exercise
Medicine
University of Bath, UK

Claire Young
Armed Forces Medic, UK

Thomas Young
Armed Forces Medic, UK

CHAPTER 1

GENERAL HISTORY AND EXAMINATION

General history

Presenting complaint(s)

⮑ How can I help you today?

History of presenting complaint(s)

⮑ When did it start? What were you doing at the time?

⮑ How did it start?

⮑ On a scale of 1 to 10 (10 being worst), how bad is it?

⮑ Is there anything that makes it worse?

⮑ Is there anything that makes it better?

⮑ Have you had this before?

⮑ Have you experienced anything else unusual?

In addition to these questions, the following chapters of this book will assist you to explore specific system presentations. Further questions relating to a general presentation of pain are included at the end of this chapter.

Past medical history

➲ Do you have any medical problems?

➲ When was this diagnosed? How severe is it? What treatment are you having?

Drug history

➲ Do you take any regular medication?

➲ Have there been any recent changes to your medication?

➲ Do you take any medication or remedies that are not prescribed?

➲ Are you allergic to any medication?

Family history

➲ Is there anyone in your family with . . .

  ● [presenting complaint]

  ● [risk factors – *see* relevant chapters]?

➲ How old were they when they were diagnosed/died?

Social history

➲ Do you live alone?

➲ Do you have any family or friends living nearby?

➲ Do you find that your [*presenting complaint*] is stopping you from doing anything, i.e. housework, gardening, job or socialising?

➲ Do you smoke? How many and for how long?

➲ Do you drink alcohol? How much and how often?

➲ Do you take any recreational drugs?

➲ Have you had any recent foreign travel?

➲ Do you have any pets?

Ideas, concerns and expectations

➲ Do you have any thoughts as to what might be causing [*presenting complaint*]?

➲ Are you worried about it or anything in particular?

➲ Is there anything specific you were hoping would happen today?

Systems review

➲ Have you ever had any fits, faints or funny turns?

➲ Do you have any problems with your ears, nose or throat?

➲ Do you ever have any difficulty breathing?

➲ Do you have a cough? Do you bring up anything and what colour is it?

➲ Do you ever have any chest pain?

➲ Do you ever experience palpitations?

➲ Have you had any changes in your bowel habit? Any changes to the stool?

➲ Do you ever have any problems passing water?

- Any burning or stinging sensation?
- Increased frequency?
- Pass a lot of water? When did this start?

➲ Do you have any problems with your joints?

➲ Has there been any unintentional weight loss?

➲ Have you had any fevers or night sweats?

➲ Have you developed any rashes?

Presentations specific to pain

There are a number of mnemonics used to structure the history of a general presentation of pain. This book will use SQITARPS as an example. If you prefer to use a different mnemonic, the questions can be rearranged accordingly.

> **SQITARPS**: **S**ite; **Q**uality; **I**ntensity; **T**iming; **A**ggravating factors; **R**elieving factors; **P**revious episodes; **S**econdary symptoms

Site

➔ Where exactly is the pain?

➔ Has the pain always been in this position? If not, where was it previously? When did it move to its current position?

➔ Does the pain move or radiate anywhere?

Quality

➔ Please describe what the pain feels like (i.e. stabbing, throbbing).

Intensity

➔ On a scale of 1 to 10, with 10 being the worst pain, where would you rate your pain?

➔ Does it stop you from doing anything?

➔ Does it wake you from your sleep?

Timing

➔ When did it start?

➔ Over what time period did the pain start (i.e. suddenly or gradually)?

➔ Is it constant?

➔ Is there a pattern? Does it come in waves?

➔ How long does it last?

Aggravating factors

➔ Is there anything that makes the pain worse?

Relieving factors

➲ Is there anything that eases the pain?

➲ Have you taken painkillers?

- Which painkillers?
- When did you take them?
- How many did you take?
- Have they worked?

Previous episodes

➲ Have you ever had this pain before?

➲ What happened then?

➲ How does this episode compare?

Secondary symptoms

➲ Have you experienced any other symptoms alongside the pain?

Chronic conditions

When taking a history from a patient with a chronic condition, it is useful to structure your history taking as follows:

1 The history of initial presenting complaint before diagnosis

2 How the complaint was diagnosed

3 Any treatment or complications after diagnosis

4 Any new problems or current concerns.

GENERAL EXAMINATION

General
- Introduction (name, grade)
- Explain examination
- Verbal consent
- Chaperone as appropriate
- Wash hands/alcohol gel
- Patient to be lying and adequately exposed.

General bedside inspection
- Obvious signs
- Body habitus
- Items around the bedside suggesting pathology.

Hands/arms
- Inspection
  - » clubbing
  - » pale palmar creases
  - » palmar erythema
  - » peripheral cyanosis
  - » cigarette staining
  - » tremor
- Palpation
  - » capillary refill
  - » pulse
    - – rate, rhythm
  - » blood pressure.

Face/neck
- Inspection
  - » pale conjunctiva

- » facies
  - – mitral; malar rash
- » hydration status
  - – sunken eyes, dry mucous membranes
- » colour
  - – pallor, jaundice, cyanosis
- » central cyanosis
- » jugular venous pressure
- » goitre
- » hirsutism
- ▶ Palpation
  - » carotids
    - – character, volume, flow
  - » lymph nodes of anterior and posterior triangles and supraclavicular fossae.

Praecordium

- ▶ Inspection
  - » scars
  - » deformities
- ▶ Palpation
  - » apex beat
- ▶ Auscultation
  - » heart sounds
  - » breath sounds.

Posterior thorax

- ▶ Auscultation
  - » breath sounds
- ▶ Palpation
  - » sacral oedema.

Abdomen

▶ Inspection
  » scars
  » swellings
▶ Palpation
  » tenderness/guarding
  » rebound tenderness
  » masses
  » hepatosplenomegaly
  » kidneys
  » bladder
▶ Percussion
  » hepatosplenomegaly
  » distended bladder
  » shifting dullness/ascites
▶ Auscultation
  » bowel sounds.

Legs/feet

▶ Inspection
  » skin changes
    – venous eczema; ulcers; varicose veins
▶ Palpation
  » pedal oedema
  » capillary refill
  » distal pulses
    – dorsalis pedis
    – posterior tibialis
  » calf tenderness.

CHAPTER 2

CARDIOVASCULAR

General

In addition to using the general history, consider the following.

Chest pain

➲ Does your chest pain radiate to your . . .
- neck
- jaw
- left/right arm
- shoulder blade?

➲ Does your chest pain get worse . . .
- on exertion
- with excitement or upset?

➲ Does it ease with . . .
- rest
- medication (glyceryl trinitrate (GTN) spray)
  - How much do you need before the pain eases?
- leaning forward?

➲ Does it occur at rest?

➲ Is it associated with . . .
- nausea/vomiting
- sweating?

Dizziness/syncope

➲ What do you mean by 'dizzy'?

➲ Does anything trigger it (e.g. standing up)?

➲ Do you experience any palpitations?

➲ Have you ever blacked out when you have become dizzy?

➲ Do you get any warning before the blackout?

➲ How long does it take before you recover?

➲ Do you feel flushed when you come round?

Dyspnoea

➲ Does it occur . . .

- on exertion
- at rest
- when lying down?

➲ How far can you walk before you feel breathless? How far could you walk . . .

- 6 months ago
- 12 months ago?

➲ Do you have a cough? Do you cough at night? Do you ever bring up anything when you cough?

➲ Do you ever wheeze?

➲ How many pillows do you use to sleep? Has this increased?

➲ Do you ever wake up in the night gasping for air?

Palpitations

➲ Do you ever feel your heart beating fast or irregularly?

➲ Can you tap out the rhythm of what it feels like?

➲ Do you have chest pain when this happens?

➲ Do you feel unwell or dizzy when this happens?

➲ How often does it happen?

➲ Is it associated with stress or anxiety?

Oedema

➲ Do you have swelling in your . . .

- ankle
- legs
- lower back?

➲ Do you feel breathless when lying down?

Risk factors

Coronary artery disease

➲ Do you smoke/have you ever smoked? How many and for how long? If you stopped smoking, when did you stop? Do you smoke anything other than tobacco?

➲ Do you exercise regularly?

➲ Do you have . . .

- diabetes
- hypertension
- high cholesterol
- familial hyperlipidaemia/high lipoprotein A?

➲ Does anyone in your family have . . .

- familial hyperlipidaemia/high lipoprotein A
- heart condition
- stroke?

CARDIOVASCULAR EXAMINATION

General

▶ Introduction (name, grade)
▶ Explain examination
▶ Verbal consent
▶ Chaperone as appropriate
▶ Wash hands/alcohol gel
▶ Patient to be lying at 45 degrees and adequately exposed.

General bedside inspection

▶ Dyspnoea
▶ Oxygen saturations, oxygen, pulse oximeter, cardiac monitor.

Hands/arms

▶ Inspection
  » clubbing; splinter haemorrhages
  » Osler's nodes; Janeway lesions
  » peripheral cyanosis
  » cigarette staining
▶ Palpation
  » capillary refill
  » pulse
    – rate, rhythm
    – collapsing pulse
    – radio-radial delay; radio-femoral delay
  » blood pressure (consider BP in both arms if radio-radial delay).

Face/neck

- Inspection
  - » pale conjunctiva
  - » xanthelasma; corneal arcus
  - » dentition; high arched palate
  - » central cyanosis
  - » jugular venous pressure
- Palpation
  - » carotids
    - – character, volume, flow.

Praecordium

- Inspection
  - » scars
  - » pacemakers
  - » deformities
- Palpation
  - » apex beat
  - » heaves and thrills
- Auscultation
  - » heart sounds
  - » areas of murmur radiation.

Posterior thorax

- Auscultation
  - » bibasal inspiratory crackles
- Palpation
  - » sacral oedema.

Legs/feet

▶ Inspection
  » skin changes
    – venous eczema; ulcers; varicose veins
▶ Palpation
  » pedal oedema
  » capillary refill
  » distal pulses
    – dorsalis pedis
    – posterior tibialis
  » calf tenderness.

Additional bedside examinations and tests

▶ Review vital signs observation chart
▶ Electrocardiogram
▶ Fundoscopy – Roth spots; signs of hypertensive retinopathy
▶ Abdominal examination – organomegaly; ascites; renal/liver bruits.

Peripheral vascular

In addition to using the general history, consider the following.

Lower limb pain

⊃ Which leg is painful?

⊃ Where exactly is it painful?

⊃ When did this problem start?

⊃ Over what time period did the pain start (suddenly or gradually)?

⊃ Does exercise precipitate it?

⊃ Does rest alleviate the pain? How long does it take?

⊃ How far can you walk before it hurts? How far could you walk . . .
  - 6 months ago
  - 12 months ago?

⊃ In the painful limb, do you also have . . .
  - swelling
  - hot joint(s)
  - varicose veins
  - heaviness or itching of legs?

Rest pain in the foot

⊃ Does this pain only occur at night?

⊃ Does hanging your foot out of bed help?

⊃ Do you have any ulcers or sores on your feet or legs?

Risk factors

Deep vein thrombosis

⊃ Have you recently had surgery?

⊃ Do you move your legs much during the day?

⊃ Has one leg been more swollen than usual?

- **Female:**
  - Are you pregnant?
  - Are you taking the combined oral contraceptive pill?
- Have you ever had a blood clot in your legs?
- Have you recently experienced a period of reduced mobility?
- Have you been unable to use any of your legs recently?
- Do you have . . .
  - cancer
  - nephrotic syndrome
  - thrombophilia?

Limb ischaemia

- Do you smoke/have you ever smoked? How many and for how long? If you stopped smoking, when did you stop? Do you smoke anything other than tobacco?
- Do you have . . .
  - diabetes
  - familial hyperlipidaemia/high lipoprotein A
  - heart disease – including atrial fibrillation
  - high cholesterol
  - hypertension?
- Does anyone in your family have . . .
  - heart disease
  - familial hyperlipidaemia/high lipoprotein A?

Varicose veins

- Have you ever had a blood clot in your legs?
- Do you stand for long periods of time?
- Female: Are you pregnant?
- Do you know what your weight is?

PERIPHERAL VASCULAR (ARTERIAL) EXAMINATION

General

- Introduction (name, grade)
- Explain examination
- Verbal consent
- Chaperone as appropriate
- Wash hands/alcohol gel
- Patient to be lying comfortably and adequately exposed.

General bedside inspection

- Cardiac monitor
- GTN spray
- Walking aid.

Inspection

- Scars
- Skin changes – shiny; thin; loss of hair; discolouration; ulceration over pressure areas.

Palpation

- Temperature
- Capillary refill
- Pulses (popliteal, posterior tibialis and dorsalis pedis)
- Buerger's test[1]
- Femoral artery and abdominal aorta.

Additional bedside examinations and tests

- Review vital signs observation chart
- Blood pressure in both arms

- Ankle brachial pressure indices
- Electrocardiogram
- Cardiovascular examination – murmurs and carotid bruits.

PERIPHERAL VASCULAR (VENOUS) EXAMINATION

General

▶ Introduction (name, grade)
▶ Explain examination
▶ Verbal consent
▶ Chaperone as appropriate
▶ Wash hands/alcohol gel
▶ Patient to be standing and adequately exposed.

General bedside inspection

▶ Body habitus
▶ Cardiac monitor
▶ GTN spray
▶ Walking aid.

Inspection

▶ Dilated/tortuous veins
▶ Erythema
▶ Venous hypertension – oedema; haemosiderin staining; lipodermatosclerosis; venous eczema; ulceration.

Palpation

▶ Thrombophlebitis
▶ Varicosities
▶ Pitting oedema
▶ Defects in deep fascia – *caution: can be painful*
▶ Saphenofemoral varix/thrill on coughing.

Special tests

▶ Trendelenburg's/tourniquet test[2]
▶ Tap test.[3]

Additional bedside examinations and tests

▶ Review vital signs observation chart
▶ Calculate body mass index
▶ Doppler ultrasound
▶ Abdominal examination.

CHAPTER 3

RESPIRATORY

In addition to using the general history, consider the following.

Breathlessness

➥ How far can you walk before you become breathless? How far could you walk . . .
  - 6 months ago
  - 12 months ago?

➥ How often are you breathless (constantly or intermittently)?

➥ How quickly does/did the breathlessness start?

➥ Does anything trigger the breathlessness?

➥ Is it associated with . . .
  - wheezing
  - rash?

Does it get worse . . .
  - on exertion
  - at night/lying flat?

➥ Have you noticed a cough, especially at night?

➥ Does it stop you from doing anything?

➥ Does anything help improve it?

➥ Do you have any leg swelling?

➥ Have you had a fever?

Chest pain

- ➲ What does the chest pain feel like (i.e. sharp, stabbing pain)?
- ➲ Does the pain go anywhere else?
- ➲ What, if anything, triggered it?
- ➲ Is it worse when breathing in?

Cough

- ➲ Does anything trigger the cough?
- ➲ Do you ever bring up anything when you cough?
  - How much and how often do you bring it up?
  - What colour is it?
  - Have you ever coughed up blood? How much and how often?
  - Do you have any trouble bringing it up?
- ➲ Do you ever wheeze?
  - How often do you wheeze (constantly or intermittently)?
  - Does anything make you wheeze?
- ➲ Have you had any cold symptoms?
- ➲ Have you travelled recently? Where?
- ➲ Have you had a fever? Is it worse at night?

Risk factors

Chronic obstructive pulmonary disease

- ➲ Do you smoke/have you ever smoked? How many and for how long? If you stopped smoking, when did you stop? Do you smoke anything other than tobacco?
- ➲ Have you or any of your family been diagnosed with an illness that may increase the risk of developing lung disease (i.e. alpha-1 antitrypsin deficiency)?

Lung cancer

⮕ Do you smoke/have you ever smoked? How many and for how long? If you stopped smoking, when did you stop? Do you smoke anything other than tobacco?

⮕ Have you ever been exposed to . . .
- asbestos
- radon
- gas
- coke?

Occupational risk factors

⮕ *Alveolitis*
- Have you ever worked in the farming industry?

⮕ *Asbestosis/Mesothelioma/lung cancer*
- Have you ever worked in the building industry?

⮕ *Asthma*
- Have you ever worked in the paint spraying or plastics industry?
- Have you ever been a solderer?

⮕ *Pneumoconiosis*
- Have you ever worked in the mining industry?

⮕ *Silicosis*
- Have you ever worked in the quarrying industry?
- Have you ever been a foundry worker?

Pneumothorax

⮕ Have you ever had a collapsed lung?

⮕ Do you have/ever had . . .
- chronic obstructive pulmonary disease
- asthma
- cystic fibrosis
- tuberculosis?

Pulmonary embolism

➲ Have you ever had a blood clot in your legs or in your lungs?

➲ Do you have any swelling in one of your legs at present?

➲ Have you had any surgery recently?

➲ Have you recently experienced a period of reduced mobility?

➲ Do you have cancer, or have you ever had cancer?

➲ Do you have a clotting disorder?

➲ Female:

- Are you pregnant?
- Are you taking the combined oral contraceptive pill?

RESPIRATORY EXAMINATION

General

▶ Introduction (name, grade)
▶ Explain examination
▶ Verbal consent
▶ Chaperone as appropriate
▶ Wash hands/alcohol gel
▶ Patient to be lying at 45 degrees and adequately exposed.

General bedside inspection

▶ Dyspnoea, accessory muscle use, chest symmetry, depth of respiration
▶ Colour (cyanosis)
▶ Cough
▶ Respiratory rate
▶ Audible wheeze
▶ Plethora, telangiectasia, oedema (superior vena cava (SVC) obstruction)
▶ Oxygen, nebuliser, inhalers, sputum pot.

Hands/arms

▶ Inspection
  » clubbing
  » peripheral cyanosis
  » cigarette staining
  » wasting of small muscles (lung cancer involving brachial plexus)
  » tremor
    – fine
    – carbon dioxide retention flap

» Palpation
  » wrist tenderness (hypertrophic pulmonary osteoarthropathy)
  » warm peripheries, dilated veins (carbon dioxide retention)
  » pulse
    – rate, rhythm
  » capillary refill time.

Face/neck

» Inspection
  » pale conjunctiva
  » signs of Horner's syndrome
  » central cyanosis
  » hydration status
  » candida/tonsillitis/pharyngitis
  » jugular venous pressure
  » engorged veins
  » tracheal tug
  » accessory muscle use
» Palpation
  » lymph nodes
  » tracheal position.

Chest (anterior followed by posterior)

» Inspection
  » shape/deformity of chest
  » scars, skin changes (bruises)
  » radiotherapy tattoos
  » prominent veins
» Palpation
  » chest expansion
  » tactile fremitus

- Percussion
  - » assess for stony dull/dull/resonant/hyper-resonance
- Auscultation
  - » vocal resonance
  - » breath sounds (vesicular or bronchial)
  - » added sounds (wheeze, crepitations).

Additional bedside examinations and tests

- Review vital signs observation chart
- Measure oxygen saturations
- Measure peak expiratory flow rate
- Assess inhaler technique
- Electrocardiogram
- Breast examination in females
- Inspect and palpate lower limbs for painful calves, oedema, heat, swelling
- Abdominal examination if malignancy suspected.

NOTES

CHAPTER 4

GASTROINTESTINAL

In addition to using the general history, consider the following.

Abdominal pain

➲ How often do you feel the pain (constantly or in waves)?

➲ Have you had any change in your bowel habit?

➲ Does it ease with . . .

- defecation
- lying still
- medication; which and how much?

➲ Have you ever had any bowel surgery?

➲ Female:

- When was your last period?
  - Are they ever painful or irregular?
- Is there any chance you may be pregnant?
- Do you have the coil fitted?
- Have you ever had a sexually transmitted infection?
- Are you known to have an ovarian cyst, endometriosis or fibroids?

Change in bowel habit

➲ How often are you opening your bowels?

➲ How often do you normally open your bowels?

- ⊃ When was the last time you opened your bowels?
- ⊃ Are you still passing wind?
- ⊃ When you open your bowels, is there any associated . . .
  - straining
  - nausea and/or vomiting
  - abdominal pain
  - bloating
  - bleeding from the back passage?
- ⊃ Do you feel constipated despite having opened your bowels?
- ⊃ How would you describe your motions? Size? Shape? Watery, loose or hard?
- ⊃ What is the colour of your stools?
- ⊃ Are they difficult to flush down the toilet?
- ⊃ Is there any blood or mucus in the stools?
- ⊃ Have you leaked any fluid or stools from your back passage?
- ⊃ Do you wake from your sleep to open your bowels?
- ⊃ Have you recently travelled abroad or been in contact with anyone with diarrhoea?
- ⊃ Have you been taking any medications (antibiotics/tablets for reflux/opioid painkillers)?

Dysphagia

- ⊃ Do you have difficulty swallowing . . .
  - liquids
  - solids?
- ⊃ At what level does food get stuck?
- ⊃ How long have you had difficulty swallowing?
- ⊃ How quickly did this problem start (suddenly or gradually)?
- ⊃ Does it happen every time you swallow?
- ⊃ Do you ever suffer with heartburn?
- ⊃ Have you unintentionally lost weight?

Jaundice

➲ Have you had any fevers?

➲ Have you been travelling recently? Where?

➲ Do you drink alcohol? On average, how much alcohol do you drink per week? For how long?

➲ Do you take any recreational drugs by injection?

➲ Have you ever had casual unprotected sex?

➲ Have you ever had a blood transfusion?

➲ Have you been in contact with jaundiced patients?

➲ Do you find your skin itches?

➲ Are you taking any medication (including non-prescription drugs)?

➲ Have you unintentionally lost weight? How much and over what time period?

➲ Has there been a change in the colour of your motions or urine?

➲ Does anyone in your family have liver disease?

➲ Do you have cancer?

Rectal bleeding

➲ When do you bleed from your back passage?

➲ How often do you bleed from your back passage?

➲ How much blood is there? Tissue only? Mixed within stools? Pan of toilet?

➲ What shade of red is the blood? Light or dark?

➲ Is there any associated rectal or abdominal pain?

➲ Do you feel a sense of urgency to open your bowels?

➲ Do you still feel the need to open your bowels despite already having done so?

➲ Have you ever had . . .
  - rectal prolapse
  - haemorrhoids
  - diverticular disease

- female only:
  - vaginal prolapse?

Vomiting

- ➲ What colour is the vomit?
  - Is there blood in the vomit? How much? How often?
- ➲ Is the vomiting worse in the morning?
- ➲ Does the vomiting occur in relation to meals?
- ➲ Is there associated abdominal pain?
- ➲ Is there recognisable food in the vomit?
- ➲ Does the vomit look as though it has coffee grounds in it?
- ➲ Is there anyone else in the household or workplace that is ill?
- ➲ What medicines are you currently taking?
- ➲ Are you opening your bowels normally?
- ➲ Are you able to pass wind?
- ➲ Have you had diarrhoea as well?

Weight loss

- ➲ How much weight have you lost and over what time period?
- ➲ Did you intend to lose weight?
- ➲ Has your appetite changed?
- ➲ Describe what food you eat during a typical day.
- ➲ Is the weight loss associated with:
  - nausea and/or vomiting
  - abdominal pain?
- ➲ Has there been a change in your bowel habit:
  - colour of motions
  - consistency of motions
  - frequency?
- ➲ Have you had a fever?

Risk factors

Cirrhosis

- ➲ Do you drink alcohol? On average, how much alcohol do you drink per week? For how long?
- ➲ Do you have . . .
  - chronic hepatitis B
  - chronic hepatitis C
  - chronic biliary disease (sclerosing cholangitis, primary biliary cirrhosis)
  - iron or copper overload
  - autoimmune hepatitis?

Dyspepsia

- ➲ Have you vomited blood?
- ➲ Have you passed any black smelly sticky stool?
- ➲ Do you smoke/have you ever smoked? How many and for how long? If you stopped smoking, when did you stop? Do you smoke anything other than tobacco?
- ➲ Do you drink alcohol? On average, how much alcohol do you drink per week? For how long?
- ➲ Do you eat spicy food regularly?
- ➲ Do you take any . . .
  - non-steroidal anti-inflammatory pain relief
  - steroids
  - bisphosphonates?
- ➲ Have you ever been treated for a *Helicobacter pylori* infection or stomach ulcer?
- ➲ Do you have a hiatus hernia?

Hepatitis B

➲ What is/was your occupation?

➲ Have you ever had a blood transfusion?

➲ Do you know if your mother had hepatitis B?

➲ Have you ever been injured from a hypodermic needle?

➲ Do you take any recreational drugs by injection?

➲ Have you ever had casual unprotected sex?

GASTROINTESTINAL EXAMINATION

General

- Introduction (name, grade)
- Explain examination
- Verbal consent
- Chaperone as appropriate
- Wash hands/alcohol gel
- Patient to be lying flat and adequately exposed.

General bedside inspection

- Jaundice
- Oedema
- Ascites
- Cachexia
- Surgical scars
- Abdominal dressings, drain, colostomy, etc.

Hands/arms

- Inspection
  - » clubbing
  - » leuconychia
  - » koilonychia
  - » palmar erythema
  - » pale palmer creases
  - » Dupuytren's contractures
  - » excoriation marks
  - » hepatic flap
- Palpation
  - » capillary refill

» pulse
  – rate, rhythm
» blood pressure.

Face/neck

▶ Inspection
  » jaundiced sclera
  » pale conjunctiva
  » Kayser–Fleischer rings of cornea
  » angular stomatitis
  » foetor hepaticus/oris
  » aphthous ulceration
  » candidiasis
  » leukoplakia
  » glossitis
▶ Palpation
  » lymph nodes
    – submental, submandibular, pre-auricular, post-auricular, anterior cervical chain, posterior cervical chain, occipital lymph nodes
    – supraclavicular fossae and axillary lymph nodes.

Chest

▶ Inspection
  » gynaecomastia
  » spider naevi.

Abdomen

▶ Inspection
  » scars
  » distension

- » prominent veins (caput medusa)
- » striae
- » obvious masses
- » visible peristalsis
- » peri-umbilical/flank haemorrhages
- Palpation (superficial and deep)
  - » tenderness
  - » rigidity
  - » masses
  - » hepatosplenomegaly
  - » ballot kidneys
  - » abdominal aortic aneurysm
- Percussion
  - » hepatosplenomegaly
  - » bladder
  - » shifting dullness/ascites
- Auscultation
  - » bowel sounds
  - » aortic, liver and renal bruits.

Additional bedside examinations and tests

- Review vital signs observation chart
- Urinalysis
- Pregnancy test in all females of reproductive age
- Digital rectal examination[4]
  - » Examine for saddle paraesthesia
- Examination of:
  - » external genitalia in the male
  - » remaining lymph nodes
  - » hernial orifices.[5]

NOTES

CHAPTER 5

ENDOCRINOLOGY

In addition to using the general history, consider the following.

Changes in facial appearance

⮑ In what ways have your facial features changed?

- staring eyes
- puffy face
- round, moon-shaped face
- widened face with more prominent features, such as forehead and jaw

⮑ Do you have any . . .

- headaches
- weight change
- palpitations
- intolerance to heat/cold
- enlarged tongue
- wide-spaced teeth
- increases in shoe or ring size?

Galactorrhoea

⮑ Female:

- Is there any chance you may be pregnant?
- Are your periods regular?

- Are you taking the combined oral contraceptive pill?

➲ Is there any associated . . .
  - visual disturbance
  - intolerance to cold
  - constipation?

➲ Are you taking . . .
  - chlorpromazine
  - metoclopramide
  - domperidone
  - antidepressants (SSRIs)?

Hoarse voice

➲ How long has your voice been hoarse?

➲ How quickly did your voice become hoarse?

➲ Is there any associated . . .
  - weight loss
  - constipation
  - dry hair and skin
  - tiredness
  - enlargement of facial features, hands and feet
  - enlarged tongue?

Hyperpigmentation

➲ Where on your body have you noticed increased pigmentation of your skin?

➲ What specifically does it look like?
  - Increased pigment over the creases on your hand and over scars
  - Thickened, pigmented and velvety lesions

➲ Is there any associated . . .
  - weight loss
  - dizziness (especially on standing)

- bruising
- weight gain
- infection one after another?

Increased thirst

⮑ Do you find you are drinking more?

⮑ Do you pass water more frequently?

⮑ Have you lost any weight recently?

⮑ Do you feel tired or lethargic?

⮑ Have you ever had problems with your kidneys?

⮑ Have you ever had a head injury?

Neck lump

⮑ What is the . . .
- size of the lump
- shape of the lump?

⮑ How long has the lump been present?

⮑ Does it affect your swallowing?

⮑ Have you ever had surgery to your neck?

⮑ Have you noticed any recent changes in . . .
- weight
- tolerance to cold/heat
- bowel habits
- pigmentation
- your heart rate?

Visual disturbance

⮑ In what way has your vision changed?

⮑ Has your colour vision changed?

⮑ Does it feel like tunnel vision?

- ➲ Is this associated with . . .
  - enlarged facial features, hands and feet?
- ➲ Is it painful?
  - Does the pain get worse with moving your eyes?
- ➲ Is this associated with . . .
  - weight loss
  - palpitations
  - agitation
  - excessive sweating
  - neck lump?

Weight gain

- ➲ How much weight have you gained and over what time period?
- ➲ Did you intend to gain weight?
- ➲ Has your appetite changed?
- ➲ Is there associated . . .
  - intolerance to cold temperatures
  - dry skin/hair
  - general tiredness/lethargy
  - constipation
  - hyperpigmentation
  - easy bruising
  - infections one after the other?

Weight loss

- ➲ How much weight have you lost?
- ➲ Over what time period have you lost this weight?
- ➲ Did you intend to lose weight?
- ➲ Has your appetite changed?
- ➲ Is there associated . . .
  - palpitations

- increased bowel habit
- excessive sweating
- increased thirst
- increased need to pass water
- general weakness
- dizziness
- hyperpigmentation?

Risk factors

Autoimmune condition

⊃ Do you or anyone in your family have . . .

- type 1 diabetes
- coeliac disease
- vitiligo
- rheumatoid arthritis
- thyroid disease
- pernicious anaemia?

Type 2 diabetes mellitus

⊃ Do you have high cholesterol?

⊃ What is your diet on a typical day?

⊃ What exercise do you do on a typical day?

⊃ Is there anyone in your family with diabetes?

⊃ Have you ever had gestational diabetes? (if appropriate)

ACROMEGALY EXAMINATION

General

- Introduction (name, grade)
- Explain examination
- Verbal consent
- Chaperone as appropriate
- Wash hands/alcohol gel
- Patient to be sitting and adequately exposed.

General bedside inspection

- Body habitus
- Hirsutism.

Hands/arms

- Inspection
  - » spade-like hands
  - » loss of thenar eminence
- Palpation
  - » pulse
    - – rate, rhythm
  - » blood pressure
  - » note hot and sweaty palms
  - » loss of sensation over thenar eminence and first three and half digits.

Face/neck

- Inspection
  - » coarse facial features
  - » prognathism
  - » forehead bossing

» enlarged tongue

» widened spaces between teeth

» acne

▶ raised jugular venous pressure.

Eyes

▶ Inspection

» prominent supra-orbital ridges

▶ Assess visual fields.

Praecordium

▶ Inspection

» scars

▶ Palpation

» apex beat

» heaves and thrills

▶ Auscultation

» heart sounds

» areas of murmur radiation.

Posterior thorax

▶ Auscultation

» basal inspiratory crackles

▶ Palpation

» sacral oedema.

Additional bedside examinations and tests

▶ Review vital signs observation chart

▶ Calculate Body Mass Index

▶ Blood sugar level

▶ Cardiovascular examination.

DIABETIC EXAMINATION

General

▸ Introduction (name, grade)

▸ Explain examination

▸ Verbal consent

▸ Chaperone as appropriate

▸ Wash hands/alcohol gel

▸ Patient to be sitting or lying and adequately exposed.

General bedside inspection

▸ Body habitus

▸ Foetor (ketosis)

▸ Blood glucose monitoring

▸ Insulin pens

▸ Fluids

▸ Insulin dextrose sliding scale

▸ Diabetic bracelet.

Hands/arms

▸ Inspection

  » peripheral cyanosis

  » cheiroarthropathy

▸ Palpation

  » pulse

    – rate, rhythm

  » blood pressure

  » distal-to-proximal vibration, temperature and fine touch sensation.

Face/neck

▶ Inspection
- » xanthelasma
- » corneal arcus
- » oral candidiasis
- » raised jugular venous pressure

▶ Palpation
- » carotids
  - – character, flow, volume.

Praecordium

▶ Auscultation
- » heart sounds.

Abdomen

▶ Inspection
- » injection sites
  - – lipohypertrophy/lipoatrophy.

Legs/feet

▶ Inspection
- » skin changes
  - – dry
  - – erythematous
  - – venous eczema
- » ulceration
- » fungal infection
- » cellulitis
- » foot deformity
- » absence of hair

- Palpation
  - » temperature changes from foot to knee
  - » peripheral pulses
    - – dorsalis pedis, posterior tibialis +/– popliteal
  - » distal-to-proximal sensation using vibration fork and monofilament, etc.

Additional bedside examinations and tests

- Review vital signs observation chart
- Calculate Body Mass Index
- Urinalysis
- Examination of cranial and peripheral nerves
- Fundoscopy
- Cardiovascular and peripheral vascular examination.

THYROID EXAMINATION

General

▹ Introduction (name, grade)
▹ Explain examination
▹ Verbal consent
▹ Chaperone as appropriate
▹ Wash hands/alcohol gel
▹ Patient to be sitting and adequately exposed.

General bedside inspection

▹ Body habitus
▹ Obvious tremor
▹ Mental state
▹ Exophthalmos
▹ Goitre/neck swelling
▹ Sweating.

Hands/arms

▹ Inspection
  » palmar erythema
  » onycholysis
  » fine tremor (exaggerated by placing paper on outstretched hands)
▹ Palpation
  » pulse
    – rate, rhythm
  » blood pressure
  » palm temperature and moisture.

Face/neck

- Inspection
  - » toad-shaped face
  - » loss of outer third eyebrows
  - » neck swelling(s)
    - – when swallowing, on tongue protrusion
  - » neck scars
- Palpation
  - » lobes of thyroid gland (size/site)
    - – when swallowing, on tongue protrusion
  - » lymph nodes of anterior and posterior triangles and supraclavicular fossae
- Percussion
  - » retrosternal goitre (from manubrium to mediastinum)
- Auscultation
  - » both lobes of gland for bruit.

Eyes

- Inspection
  - » exophthalmos, lid retraction, proptosis
  - » conjunctival oedema
- Eye movements
  - » ask about pain and diplopia
  - » lid lag
- Visual acuity of each eye via Snellen chart
- Colour vision via Ishihara chart.

Legs

- Inspection
  - » pretibial myxoedema

- Reflexes
  - » Proximal myopathy.

Additional bedside examinations and tests
- Review vital signs observation chart
- Calculate Body Mass Index
- Fundoscopy.

NOTES

CHAPTER 6

HAEMATOLOGY

In addition to using the general history, consider the following.

Anaemia

➲ Do you find that you have been feeling more tired than usual?
➲ Have you experienced any . . .
  • chest pain
  • palpitations
  • shortness of breath
  • dizzy spells
  • ankle swelling?

Bleeding

➲ Do you bruise easily? Is this recent or longstanding? Do you sometimes bruise without any obvious reason?
➲ Have you noticed any small red/purple spots on your skin?
➲ Have you experienced any nosebleeds? If so, from one or both nostrils?
➲ Have you experienced bleeding from the gums?
➲ If you cut yourself, how long does it take for you to stop bleeding?
➲ Female: Do you experience heavy periods? If so, how many days do you have heavy bleeding? Do you pass clots?
➲ Is there any joint pain or swelling?

Infection

⮑ Have you been travelling recently?

⮑ Have you ever had infections one after the other?

⮑ How many infections have you had in the last 6 months? How many of these required antibiotics?

⮑ Have you ever required hospital treatment for infections?

⮑ Have you had infections you have not been able to clear properly?

⮑ Have you experienced any . . .

- fever
- shaking
- night sweats
- weight loss?

HAEMATOLOGICAL EXAMINATION

General

- Introduction (name, grade)
- Explain examination
- Verbal consent
- Chaperone as appropriate
- Wash hands/alcohol gel
- Patient to be sitting or lying adequately exposed.

General bedside inspection

- General pallor
- Obvious superficial bruising, petechiae and/or purpura
- Obvious lumps and bumps
- Obvious large joint swelling.

Inspection

- Clubbing
- Koilonychia
- Onycholysis
- Knuckle hyperpigmentation
- Pale conjunctiva and tongue
- Angular stomatitis
- Glossitis
- Features of congestive heart failure.

Palpation

- Pulse
  - » rate, rhythm
- Blood pressure

- Lymphadenopathy
  - » neck
  - » axillae
  - » inguinal region
- Hepatosplenomegaly
- Bony tenderness
  - » spine
  - » sternum
  - » clavicles
  - » shoulders.

Additional bedside examinations and tests

- Review vital signs observation chart.

CHAPTER 7

RENAL

In addition to using the general history, consider the following.

Dysuria

➲ Does it sting or burn when you pass water?

➲ How long has it felt like this?

➲ Is there any associated . . .

- blood

- fever

- pain in the lower abdomen or side

- discharge?

➲ Have you had this before? How many times?

Loin pain

➲ How quickly did the pain start (suddenly or gradually)?

➲ Does it come in waves or is it constant?

➲ Does the pain radiate anywhere?

➲ Is there any associated . . .

- burning or stinging sensation when passing water

- increased amount of water being passed

- nausea/vomiting

- fever?

➲ Any change in bowel habit?

Nocturia

➲ How often do you pass water in the night?

➲ Do you experience a sudden urge to pass water?

➲ Are you passing water more often than usual?

➲ Do you have any . . .

- rashes
- joint pain
- frequent nosebleeds
- hearing loss?

➲ Male:

- Does it take some time before you begin to pass water?
- Have you noticed a poor stream when passing water?
- Do you ever leak after passing water?

➲ Females who are pregnant:

- Do you experience headaches with associated visual disturbance?
- What was your last blood pressure reading?

Visual haematuria

➲ How long have you noticed blood in your urine?

➲ Is it at the beginning or end of your stream?

➲ Are there any blood clots?

➲ Is it painful to pass water?

➲ Have you unintentionally lost weight recently?

➲ Do you feel tired or lethargic?

➲ Is there any associated . . .

- swelling around the eyes and ankles
- difficulty breathing
- nausea/vomiting
- fever
- change in frequency of passing water?

Risk factors

Acute kidney injury

⮕ Have you passed blood in either your stools or vomit?

⮕ Are you currently experiencing diarrhoea and vomiting?

⮕ Are you taking any new medication, such as blood pressure medication or anti-inflammatory pain relief?

⮕ Have you noticed any blood in your urine?

⮕ Have you unintentionally lost weight?

⮕ Male:

- Does it take some time before you begin to pass water?
- Have you noticed a poor stream when passing water?
- Do you ever leak after passing water?

Chronic kidney disease

⮕ Do you have . . .

- diabetes
- high blood pressure?

⮕ Does anyone in your family have . . .

- polycystic kidneys
- renal disease?

Glomerulonephritis

⮕ Have you had pharyngitis over the past few weeks?

⮕ Do you have . . .

- cancer
- diabetes
- high blood pressure
- rheumatoid arthritis
- systemic lupus erythematosus
- vasculitic disease (i.e. Wegener's granulomatosis, Henoch–Schönlein purpura)?

⊃ Have you had any antibiotics recently? Which and what were they for?

⊃ Female: Are you pregnant?

⊃ Have you recently changed sexual partner?

⊃ When did you last have sexual intercourse?

Pyelonephritis (chronic)

⊃ Did you have any urine infections as a child?

⊃ Does anyone in your family have kidney disease?

⊃ Have you ever had . . .

- renal or pelvic surgery
- renal stones
- recurrent urine infections?

Renal calculi

⊃ How much water do you drink in a typical day?

⊃ Are you taking any medication such as diuretics/water tablets?

⊃ Do you have or have you ever had . . .

- gout
- metabolic disease
- kidney stones
- renal tract abnormality?

⊃ Does anyone in your family have kidney stones?

Tubulointerstitial nephritis

⊃ Are you taking any . . .

- prescribed medication (i.e. NSAIDs, lithium, probenecid)
- over-the-counter medication (i.e. NSAIDs)
- herbal remedies?

⊃ Do you have any back aches/tenderness?

UTI/acute pyelonephritis

➲ How much water do you drink in a typical day?

➲ Have you been immobile or unable to get to a toilet to pass water recently?

➲ Do you have . . .

- diabetes
- renal tract abnormality?

RENAL EXAMINATION

General

- Introduction (name, grade)
- Explain examination
- Verbal consent
- Chaperone as appropriate
- Wash hands/alcohol gel
- Patient to be lying flat and adequately exposed.

General bedside inspection

- Pallor
- Tetany/myoclonus
- Oedema
- Signs of dehydration
- Signs of dialysis access.

Hands/arms

- Inspection
  - » leuconychia
  - » Beau's lines
  - » Muehrcke's lines
  - » pale palmar creases
  - » bruising
  - » excoriation marks
  - » arteriovenous fistula
  - » gouty tophi
- Palpation
  - » arteriovenous fistula
  - » pulse
    - – rate, rhythm

» blood pressure

▶ Auscultation

» arteriovenous fistula.

Face/neck

▶ Inspection

» jaundiced sclera

» pale conjunctiva

» uraemic foetor

» band keratopathy

» dry mucous membranes

» aphthous ulceration

» jugular venous pressure.

Chest

▶ Auscultation

» bibasal crepitation.

Abdomen

▶ Inspection

» scar

  – nephrectomy

  – peritoneal dialysis

  – masses

  – ectopic kidney

» ascites

▶ Palpation (superficial and deep)

» masses

» ballot kidneys

» bladder

- Percussion
  - » bladder
  - » shifting dullness/ascites
- Auscultation
  - » renal bruit.

Legs

- Inspection
  - » oedema
- Palpation
  - » peripheral neuropathy.

Additional bedside examinations and tests

- Review vital signs observation chart
- Urinalysis
- Fundoscopy
- Male: Digital rectal examination for enlarged prostate[4]
- Female: Vaginal examination for prolapse. As per Chapter 12 on gynaecology.

CHAPTER 8

NEUROLOGY

Cranial nerves

In addition to using the general history, consider the following.

Change in higher cortical functioning

⮀ Are you right or left-handed?

⮀ Has there been a change in your memory or ability to concentrate?

⮀ Do you have difficulty finding the right words in conversation?

⮀ Have you ever become lost while travelling along a familiar route?

⮀ Do you have difficulty dressing?

⮀ Has there been a change in your mood?

Diplopia

⮀ Do images appear side by side or on top of each other?

⮀ Is it relieved by covering one or the other eye?

⮀ Does it get worse when you look in a particular direction?

⮀ Is it constant?

Dizziness

⮀ What do you mean by 'dizzy/vertigo/spinning'?

⮀ Does it feel as though you are spinning? Does it feel as though the room is spinning?

⮀ Has this affected your balance?

- How long does it last?
- Do you feel sick when it happens? Have you vomited?
- Is it better or worse when your eyes are open?
- Do you experience any high-pitched ringing in your ear(s)?
- Have you had any hearing loss?
- Do you feel as though your ear feels full?
- Is it triggered by different movements or head positions?
- Have you ever had ear problems or surgery?

Dysphasia

- Have you or anyone else noticed a change in your speech (i.e. slurred)?
- Do people always understand what you are saying?
- Do you find it difficult to find the right words?
- Do you ever experience drooling of saliva?

Facial weakness

- Can you raise both eyebrows?
- Do you find that saliva comes out of your mouth without you realising?
- Is there a loss of taste on the front part of your tongue?
- Do noises appear excessively loud in any ear? Which ear?
- Does your eye on that side still water?

Headaches

- What does it feel like (i.e. tight band, sharp stabbing, throbbing, like a blow to the head)?
- Can you point to where it is?
- Is it on one side?

⮞ Any associated . . .
- visual disturbance before or during the headache
- scalp tenderness
- eye pain
- sensitivity to light
- neck stiffness
- nausea or vomiting
- limb weakness
- limb numbness/tingling?

⮞ Do you know of anything that may trigger it (i.e. food, alcohol, stress)?

⮞ Is it worse . . .
- in the morning
- when coughing, sneezing, straining or lying down?

⮞ How does this headache differ from others you have had?

Seizure

⮞ Was anyone with you at the time of the seizure?

⮞ What is the last thing you remember before the seizure?

⮞ Did you feel it coming on? How did it feel?

⮞ Do you know of anything that may have triggered it?

⮞ Have you had any recent head or neck injury?

⮞ Do you remember what happened during the seizure?

⮞ Did you . . .
- lose control of your bladder or bowels
- bite your tongue?

⮞ After the seizure, did you feel . . .
- confused
- tired?

⮞ Have you ever had a seizure before?

⮞ Have you been diagnosed with epilepsy?

⮕ Does anyone in your family have epilepsy?

⮕ Do you drink alcohol? On average, how much alcohol do you drink per week? For how long? Have you drunk alcohol recently?

⮕ Do you take any recreational drugs?

Visual disturbances

⮕ Have you noticed any change or loss in your vision?

⮕ Which eye is affected?

⮕ To what extent is the visual loss (complete or partial)?

- If partial, where in your visual field is affected (central or peripheral)?

⮕ How quickly did this problem start (suddenly or gradually)?

⮕ Was it similar to a black curtain or veil coming across your eye?

⮕ Have you noticed a change in your colour vision (i.e. red colour vision)?

Risk factors

Cerebral haemorrhage

⮕ Have you suffered a recent head injury?

⮕ Are you taking anti-coagulants (warfarin, clopidogrel)?

⮕ Do you have . . .

- high blood pressure
- a known medical condition of the brain
- bleeding disorders
- brain tumours?

⮕ Does anyone in your family have . . .

- high blood pressure
- a known medical condition of the brain
- bleeding disorders
- brain tumours?

Cerebral infarction

➲ Do you have . . .
- high blood pressure
- diabetes mellitus
- cardiac disease (including atrial fibrillation)
- blood clotting disorder
- cancer?

➲ Do you smoke/have you ever smoked? How many and for how long? If you stopped smoking, when did you stop? Do you smoke anything other than tobacco?

➲ Do you take recreational drugs?

➲ Female: Do you take the combined oral contraceptive pill?

Epilepsy

➲ Have you suffered a recent head injury?

➲ Do you have or have you ever had . . .
- Alzheimer's disease
- intracranial tumour or any other cancer
- stroke
- prolonged febrile convulsions as a child
- meningitis
- encephalitis?

Migraines

➲ Does anyone in your family experience migraines?

➲ Do you take . . .
- anticoagulants
- painkillers?

➲ Female: Do you take the combined oral contraceptive pill?

CRANIAL NERVE EXAMINATION

General

▶ Introduction (name, grade)

▶ Explain examination

▶ Verbal consent

▶ Chaperone as appropriate

▶ Wash hands/alcohol gel

▶ Patient to be sitting.

General bedside inspection

▶ Strabismus

▶ Ptosis

▶ Facial drooping

▶ Drooling.

CN I (Olfactory)

▶ Ask if patient has had a change in their sense of smell.

CN II (Optic)

▶ Visual acuity of each eye via Snellen chart

▶ Colour vision via Ishihara chart

▶ Visual fields

▶ Direct and indirect consensual light reflex (also assesses CN III)

▶ Swinging light reflex

▶ Accommodation

▶ Fundoscopy.

CN III, IV, VI (Oculomotor, Trochlear, Abducent)

- Eye movements
  - » Ask about double vision (horizontal or vertical)
  - » Assess for nystagmus.

CN V (Trigeminal)

- Palpation
  - » Muscles of mastication (masseter and temporalis)
  - » Sensation of ophthalmic, maxillary and mandibular divisions
  - » Corneal reflex if necessary
  - » Jaw reflex.

CN VII (Facial)

- Ask patient if they have noticed any change in taste
- Inspection
  - » vesicles around external auditory meatus
- Palpation
  - » frontalis (raise eyebrows against resistance)
  - » orbicularis oculi (eyes screwed up)
  - » buccinator (puff out cheeks against resistance)
  - » orbicularis oris (smile showing teeth)
  - » platysma (tense neck).

CN VIII (Vestibulocochlear)

- Whisper in each ear and ask patient to repeat what they hear
- Rinne's test[6]
- Weber's test.[7]

CN IX (Glossopharyngeal)

- Gag reflex if necessary (also assesses CN X).

CN X (Vagus)

- Ensure patient has no swallowing difficulties then ask patient to swallow
- Inspection
  - » deviation of uvula as patient says, 'Ahh'.

CN XI (Accessory)

- Inspection
  - » trapezius (shrug shoulders against resistance)
  - » sternocleidomastoids (turning head against resistance).

CN XII (Hypoglossal)

- Inspection
  - » protruded tongue
  - » fasciculation
  - » deviation.

Additional bedside examinations and tests

- Review vital signs observation chart.

Peripheral neurology

In addition to using the general history, consider the following.

Muscle weakness

➲ Where is the muscle weakness? Is it confined to . . .
  - one limb
  - one side of the body
  - the extremities only (i.e. feet and/or hands)?

➲ Is it constant? Does it fluctuate?

➲ Is the weakness accompanied by stiffness or is it floppy?

➲ How quickly did the problem start (suddenly or gradually)?

➲ Does it feel as though your body is wrapped in bandages?

Sensory disturbance

➲ What does it feel like (i.e. numb, tingling, pain)?

➲ Where precisely is the sensory disturbance?

➲ Does the sensory disturbance affect your abdomen or chest area?

Tremor

➲ Is the tremor mainly . . .
  - at rest
  - when your hands are held out
  - when you use your hands?

➲ Is the tremor relieved by alcohol?

➲ Is there a family history of tremor?

Risk factors

Cerebral haemorrhage

➲ As per Cranial Nerve section.

Cerebral infarction

➲ As per Cranial Nerve section.

UPPER LIMB EXAMINATION

General

- Introduction (name, grade)
- Explain examination
- Verbal consent
- Chaperone as appropriate
- Wash hands/alcohol gel
- Patient to be lying and adequately exposed.

General bedside inspection

- General posture
- Muscle atrophy
- Fasciculation
- Contracture
- Abnormal movement
- Tremor.

Tone

- Assess tone of upper arms and arms
  - » rigidity (i.e. cogwheel/clasp knife)
  - » spasticity (pronator drift)
  - » flaccidity.

Power

- Assess muscle power against resistance
  - » abduct and adduct arms (C5)
  - » flex and extend arms (C6; C7)
  - » flex and extend wrists (C6; C7)
  - » flex and extend fingers (C8; T1)
  - » abduct and adduct fingers (C8; T1).

Sensation

▶ Assess light touch, pain, temperature and vibration sense
  » tip of shoulder (C4)
  » lateral surface of upper arm (C5)
  » thumb (C6)
  » middle finger (C7)
  » little finger (C8)
  » medial epicondyle of elbow (T1)
  » medial surface of upper arm (T2).

Reflexes

▶ Assess reflexes of upper limb
  » biceps (C5, C6)
  » triceps (C6, C7)
  » supinator (C5, C6).

Coordination

▶ Inspection
  » dysdiadochokinesis
  » past pointing.

Proprioception

▶ Assess proprioception of index finger.

Additional bedside examinations and tests

▶ Review vital signs observation chart.

LOWER LIMB EXAMINATION

General

▶ Introduction (name, grade)

▶ Explain examination

▶ Verbal consent

▶ Chaperone as appropriate

▶ Wash hands/alcohol gel

▶ Patient to be lying and adequately exposed.

General bedside inspection

▶ General posture

▶ Muscle atrophy

▶ Fasciculation

▶ Contracture

▶ Abnormal movement

▶ Tremor.

Tone

▶ Assess tone of thighs and legs
  » rigidity
  » spasticity
  » flaccidity

▶ Clonus.

Power

▶ Assess muscle power against resistance
  » flex and extend the hip (L2, S1)
  » flex and extend the knee (S2, L3)
  » foot dorsiflexion and plantarflexion (L4, S1)
  » toe dorsiflexion and plantarflexion (L5).

Sensation

▶ Assess light touch, pain, temperature and vibration sense
  » anterior surface of thigh (L2)
  » knee (L3)
  » medial surface of leg (L4)
  » lateral surface of leg (L5)
  » lateral surface of little toe (S1)
▶ Assess for saddle paraesthesia.

Reflexes

▶ Assess reflexes of lower limb
  » knee (L3, L4)
  » ankle (S1)
  » Babinski reflex.

Coordination

▶ Inspection
  » heel–shin test.

Proprioception

▶ Assess proprioception of big toe.

Additional bedside examinations and tests

▶ Review vital signs observation chart
▶ Assess gait
▶ Romberg's test[8]
▶ Digital rectal examination[4] if spinal cord injury suspected.

NOTES

CHAPTER 9

EAR, NOSE AND THROAT

In addition to using the general history, consider the following.

Generic questions as part of all ENT histories

➲ Do you, or have you . . .
- coughed up any blood
- vomited any blood
- had any nosebleeds
- had any bleeding from the ears
- have any facial weakness?

General

Face pain

➲ Does the pain get worse . . .
- when leaning forward
- to touch?
➲ Does your jaw ache on eating?
➲ Is it associated with a blocked/runny nose?
➲ Do you have any dental problems?

● Do you have . . .
  - polymyalgia rheumatica
  - migraines?

Ears

Hearing loss

● How long have you noticed a hearing loss?

● To what extent is the hearing loss (partial or complete)?

● Are both ears affected or just one?

● Does anyone in your family have hearing problems?

● Have you had an injury or surgery to your ears?

● Have you been treated for any serious illness such as tuberculosis or septicaemia (ototoxic drugs)?

● Have you been exposed to a loud noise for any length of time?

● Is there any associated . . .
  - vertigo
  - high-pitched ringing in the ear?

Otalgia

● Is the pain on the outside or inside of your ear?

● Is there any discharge?

● Have you placed anything into your ear that may still be there?

● Do you feel generally unwell?

● Have you ever had an ear operation?

● Have you ever had your ears syringed?

● Do you use cotton buds?

● Have you hurt your ear recently?

● Have you been swimming or on an aeroplane recently?

● Has your hearing been affected?

Vertigo

⮁ What do you mean by 'dizzy/vertigo/spinning'?

⮁ Does it feel as though you are spinning? Does it feel as though the room is spinning?

⮁ Has this affected your balance?

⮁ How long does it last?

⮁ Do you feel sick when it happens?

⮁ Do you experience any high-pitched ringing in your ear(s)?

⮁ Has there been any hearing loss?

⮁ Do you feel as though your ear feels full?

⮁ Is it triggered by certain movements or positions of your head?

⮁ Have you ever had ear problems or ear surgery?

EAR EXAMINATION

General

- Introduction (name, grade)
- Explain examination
- Verbal consent
- Chaperone as appropriate
- Wash hands/alcohol gel
- Patient to be sitting.

General bedside inspection

- Patient discomfort/pain
- Obvious deformity.

Hearing

- Rinne's test[6]
- Weber's test.[7]

Inspection

- Examine good/better ear first; inspect for scars, skin changes, discharge
  - » pinna
  - » external auditory meatus
  - » mastoid bone.

Palpation

- Tragus
  - » tenderness
  - » perilymph fistula
- Ear lobe
  - » tenderness on pulling.

Otoscope

- Inspection
  - » canal
    - – wax
    - – inflammation
    - – discharge
  - » tympanic membrane
    - – colour
    - – malleus
    - – protrusion
    - – retraction pockets
    - – perforation
    - – discharge
    - – blood
    - – cholesteatoma.

Additional bedside examinations and tests

- Review vital signs observation chart
- Romberg's[8] and Unterberger's[9] tests
- Head and neck examination
- Cranial nerve examination
- Audiometry and tympanography
- Full nose and throat examinations.

Nose

Blocked nose

➲ Is the nose blocked/runny constantly or only some of the time (day or night)?

➲ Have you placed anything up your nose that may still be there?

➲ Does it vary with the seasons?

➲ Have you had a change in your sense of smell?

➲ Is there any associated nasal discharge?

➲ Which nostril is affected?

➲ Do you have . . .

● asthma

● any allergies?

➲ Do you sniff glue or illicit substances (e.g. cocaine)?

Risk factors

Rhinosinusitis

➲ Do you have . . .

● asthma

● eczema

● hay fever

● cystic fibrosis?

➲ Does anyone in your family have . . .

● rhinosinusitis

● asthma

● eczema

● hay fever

● cystic fibrosis?

NOSE EXAMINATION

General

- Introduction (name, grade)
- Explain examination
- Verbal consent
- Chaperone as appropriate
- Wash hands/alcohol gel
- Patient to be sitting.

General bedside inspection

- Deviation from midline
- Saddle deformity
- Crusting of nostrils.

Palpation

- Tenderness over the nasal bridge.

Inspection with nasal speculum

- Patency
- Septal defects (deviation, haematoma, perforation)
- Obstruction.

Additional bedside examinations and tests

- Review vital signs observation chart
- Nasal endoscopy.

Throat

Hoarse voice

- ➲ Have you had a recent cold?
- ➲ Do you smoke/have you ever smoked? How many and for how long? If you stopped smoking, when did you stop? Do you smoke anything other than tobacco?
- ➲ Do you drink alcohol? On average, how much alcohol do you drink per week? For how long?
- ➲ Do you have thyroid problems?
- ➲ Have you had any recent neck surgery?
- ➲ Have you ever had cancer?
- ➲ What type of work do you do?
- ➲ Have you abused your voice, i.e. shouting, singing?

Lump in the neck

- ➲ How long has it been present?
- ➲ Has the lump changed in size?
- ➲ Is the lump painful?
- ➲ Do you sweat at night?
- ➲ Have you unintentionally lost weight recently?
- ➲ Do you have thyroid problems?
- ➲ Do you have a cough?
- ➲ Have you had any discharge from your nose?
- ➲ Are you generally well?
- ➲ Have you noticed any lumps anywhere else?

Lump in the throat

- ➲ How quickly did this problem start (suddenly or gradually)?
- ➲ Have you swallowed anything that may have lodged in your throat?
- ➲ Is it difficult to swallow?

➲ Is it painful to swallow?

➲ Do you feel generally unwell with it?

➲ Have you experienced any unintentional weight loss?

➲ Do you find it difficult to keep your breath fresh?

➲ Do you experience a gargling sensation in your throat?

➲ Do you have recurrent coughs or chest infections?

➲ Are you under more stress than usual?

Sore mouth or throat

➲ Have you had a fever or felt generally unwell?

➲ Do you have a lump sensation in your throat?

➲ Is it painful to swallow?

➲ Do you experience heartburn or indigestion?

Risk factors

Carcinoma of the oral cavity, oropharynx and larynx

➲ What ethnicity are you?

➲ Do you smoke/have you ever smoked? How many and for how
long? If you stopped smoking, when did you stop? Do you smoke
anything other than tobacco?

➲ Do you drink alcohol? On average, how much alcohol do you drink
per week? For how long?

➲ Do you have any dental problems?

➲ Do you have a sensitivity to aspirin?

THROAT EXAMINATION

General

▶ Introduction (name, grade)

▶ Explain examination

▶ Verbal consent

▶ Chaperone as appropriate

▶ Wash hands/alcohol gel

▶ Patient to be sitting.

General bedside inspection

▶ Lumps/swellings in neck

   » in normal anatomical position

   » with the tongue protruding

   » while swallowing water.

Palpation

▶ Lobes of thyroid gland

   » in the normal anatomical position

   » with the tongue protruding

   » while swallowing water

▶ Lymph nodes of anterior and posterior triangles and supraclavicular fossae.

Inspection

▶ Mouth

   » lips and teeth

   » superior, posterior and lateral surfaces of tongue

   » buccal mucosa

   » hard and soft palate

   » uvula

- » anterior and posterior pillars
- » palatine tonsils
- » oropharynx.

Additional bedside examinations and tests

- ▶ Review vital signs observation chart
- ▶ Facial nerve examination.

NOTES

CHAPTER 10

OPHTHALMOLOGY

In addition to using the general history, consider the following.

Diplopia

➲ Do images appear side by side or on top of each other?

➲ Is it relieved by covering one or the other eye?

➲ Does it get worse when you look in a particular direction?

Gradual visual loss

➲ Is it in one eye or both eyes?

➲ To what extent is the visual loss?

➲ Where in your field of vision is it lost?

➲ Do images appear distorted?

➲ Does your vision appear cloudy or blurry?

➲ Is there a change in colour vision (more brown–yellow)?

➲ Do you have . . .

- diabetes
- hypertension?

Red eye

➲ Is it one eye or both eyes?

➲ Is your vision affected?

➲ Can you see halos around objects?

- ⮑ Is it painful?
- ⮑ Is there a gritty or foreign body sensation?
- ⮑ Is there any pus or watery discharge?
- ⮑ Are your eyes sensitive to light?
- ⮑ Do you feel generally unwell? Any nausea and/or vomiting?
- ⮑ Did anything precede it (bright light, darkness)?
- ⮑ Any previous injury or trauma?
- ⮑ Do you wear contact lenses?

Sudden visual loss

- ⮑ Is it painful?
- ⮑ Have you recently been experiencing . . .
  - headaches
  - scalp tenderness
  - jaw pain when eating?
- ⮑ Do you feel generally unwell (fever, nausea/vomiting)?
- ⮑ To what extent is the visual loss?
- ⮑ Is the visual loss intermittent?
- ⮑ Is there a shadow or veil covering any part of your vision?
- ⮑ Was there a sudden appearance of floaters or persistent flashing lights?
- ⮑ Have you noticed a change in your colour vision (red colour vision)?
- ⮑ Do you have . . .
  - diabetes
  - high blood pressure
  - heart disease (including atrial fibrillation)
  - multiple sclerosis?

Risk factors

Age-related macular degeneration

➲ How old are you?

➲ Do you smoke/have you ever smoked? How many and for how long? If you stopped smoking, when did you stop? Do you smoke anything other than tobacco?

➲ Does anyone in your family have age-related macular degeneration?

➲ Do you have any heart conditions?

Cataracts

➲ Do you take steroid medication?

➲ How old are you?

➲ Do you have . . .
- diabetes
- rheumatoid arthritis?

➲ Do you smoke/have you ever smoked? How many and for how long? If you stopped smoking, when did you stop? Do you smoke anything other than tobacco?

Primary open angle glaucoma

➲ Does anyone in your family have primary open angle glaucoma?

➲ What ethnicity are you?

➲ How old are you?

Uveitis

➲ Do you have . . .
- inflammatory arthritis (i.e. rheumatoid arthritis, ankylosing spondylitis)
- inflammatory bowel disease
- sarcoidosis?

OPHTHALMOLOGICAL EXAMINATION

General

▮ Introduction (name, grade)

▮ Explain examination

▮ Verbal consent

▮ Chaperone as appropriate

▮ Wash hands/alcohol gel

▮ Patient to be sitting. Glasses/contact lenses removed.

General bedside inspection

▮ Inspection
  » surrounding skin
    – vesicles
  » strabismus
  » pupil size and shape
  » ptosis
  » entropion/ectropion
  » proptosis
  » discharge
  » conjunctiva
  » redness
  » chemosis
  » cornea
    – corneal opacity
    – corneal abrasion – requires fluorescein staining
    – dendritic ulcer – requires fluorescein staining
  » sclera
    – injection
    – jaundice

» orbit and eyeballs
  - deformity
  - foreign body
  - fluid level in anterior chamber.

Assessment
▶ Visual acuity of each eye via Snellen chart (with and without pinhole)
▶ Colour vision using Ishihara chart
▶ Visual fields (confrontation testing)
▶ Direct and indirect consensual light reflex
▶ Swinging light reflex
▶ Accommodation
▶ Eye movements.

Fundoscopy
▶ Inspection
  » Red reflex
  » Retina
  » Blood vessels
  » Optic disc
  » Macula.

NOTES

CHAPTER 11

GENITOURINARY

Male genitourinary

In addition to using the general history, consider the following.

Incontinence

➲ Do you feel an urge to pass water before you do pass water?

➲ Do you get warning before passing water?

➲ Is it painful to pass water?

➲ Have you felt unwell lately?

➲ Do you wet yourself at night?

➲ Do you have backache?

➲ Are your legs weaker than usual?

➲ Do you ever lose control of your bowels?

➲ Do you have any numbness around your back passage?

➲ Have you unintentionally lost weight?

Infertility

➲ How long have you and your partner been trying to conceive?

➲ Are you having regular sex?

➲ Do either you or your partner have children?

➲ Do you have difficulty obtaining or maintaining an erection?

➲ Do you ejaculate?

➲ Do you understand the timing of ovulation in your partner?

- Are you on any medication such as sulfasalazine?
- Do you have diabetes?

Retention

- When passing water, does it . . .
  - take a while to start
  - stop and start
  - dribble?
- Do you have any associated . . .
  - pain on passing water
  - abdominal pain
  - abdominal swelling?
- Have you experienced any leakage?
- Is this the first time this has happened?
- Have you ever required a catheter for retention?
- Do you have backache?
- Have you unintentionally lost weight?

Skin lesion(s)

- How many lesions are there?
- Where exactly is it/are they?
- Is it/are they painful?
- What do they look like (ulcer, wart)?
- Do they discharge?
- Have you had a recent change of sexual partner?
- Have you ever had unprotected sex?
- Do you feel generally unwell? Feverish?
- Are there any lumps in your groin?

Testicular pain

- How quickly did the pain start (suddenly or gradually)?

- When did the pain start?
- Was the pain preceded by trauma?
- Was the pain preceded by a fever or swelling of the salivary glands (mumps)?
- Was the pain preceded by burning on passing water or discharge?
- Is your scrotum swollen?

Urethral discharge

- What colour is the discharge?
- Is there any blood in the discharge?
- Any problems passing urine? Burning, stinging?
- Have you recently had unprotected sex?
- Have you recently changed sexual partners?
- How many sexual partners have you had over the past 12 months?
- Does your partner complain of discharge?
- Have you experienced . . .
  - eye pain, redness, discharge or grittiness
  - painful joints
  - recent gastroenteritis?
- Do you have diabetes?
- Have you taken any antibiotics recently?

Risk factors

Sexually transmitted infections

- Have you recently changed sexual partner?
- How many sexual partners have you had over the past 12 months?
- Have you ever had unprotected sex?
- Have you ever had or do you have a sexually transmitted infection?
- Has any partner(s) been treated for a sexually transmitted infection?

MALE GENITOURINARY EXAMINATION

General

▶ Introduction (name, grade)

▶ Explain examination

▶ Verbal consent

▶ Chaperone as appropriate

▶ Wash hands/alcohol gel

▶ Wear gloves

▶ Patient to be lying and adequately exposed.

General bedside inspection

▶ Patient discomfort or pain

▶ Distribution of facial, axillary and abdominal hair

▶ Gynaecomastia.

Groin

▶ Inspection

  » swelling

  » erythema of creases

  » sinuses

  » fistulae

▶ Palpation

  » superficial and deep inguinal lymph nodes.

Scrotum

▶ Inspection

  » asymmetry

  » swelling

▶ Palpation (one testis at a time)

  » testes, epididymis, vas deferens

- size
- consistency
- tenderness
▶ Perform
  » transillumination
  » cremasteric reflex.

Penis and urethral meatus
▶ Inspection (retract foreskin to expose glans penis)
  » abnormalities
  » discharge.

Additional bedside examinations and tests
▶ Review vital signs observation chart
▶ Urethral swab
▶ Urine sample
▶ Fundoscopy
▶ Abdominal examination
▶ Hernial orifice examination.[5]

Female genitourinary

In addition to using the general history, consider the following.

Skin lesions

- ⊃ How many lesions are there?
- ⊃ Is it/are they painful?
- ⊃ What do they look like (ulcer, wart)?
- ⊃ Do they discharge?
- ⊃ Have you changed your sexual partner recently?
- ⊃ Have you ever had unprotected sex?
- ⊃ Do you feel generally unwell? Feverish?
- ⊃ Are there any lumps in your groin?

Vaginal discharge

- ⊃ What colour is the discharge?
- ⊃ Is it thin and watery or thick?
- ⊃ Does it smell offensive (i.e. fishy)?
- ⊃ Is there any associated . . .
  - pain or irritation of the surrounding area
  - pain on intercourse
  - skin lesions?
- ⊃ Have you been on any antibiotics recently?
- ⊃ Do you have diabetes?
- ⊃ Do you have any allergies?
- ⊃ Has anything preceded it (i.e. sex, change of washing powder/ soap)?
- ⊃ Have you recently changed sexual partners?
- ⊃ How many sexual partners have you had over the past 12 months?
- ⊃ Have you ever had unprotected sex?

Vulval irritation

⮑ Do you suffer from any skin conditions?

⮑ Has anything triggered it (i.e. change in soap or washing powder)?

⮑ Do you have any allergies?

⮑ Do you have any associated . . .

- discharge
- skin lesions?

Risk factors

Sexually transmitted infections

⮑ Have you recently changed sexual partner?

⮑ How many sexual partners have you had over the past 12 months?

⮑ Have you ever had unprotected sex?

⮑ Do you live in a metropolitan area?

⮑ Have you ever had or do you have a sexually transmitted infection?

⮑ Has any partner(s) been treated for a sexually transmitted infection?

FEMALE GENITOURINARY EXAMINATION

General

- Introduction (name, grade)
- Explain examination
- Verbal consent
- Chaperone as appropriate
- Wash hands/alcohol gel
- Wear gloves
- Patient to be lying and adequately exposed.

General bedside inspection

- Patient discomfort or pain.

Groin

- Inspection
  » erythema
  » swelling
  » ulceration
  » sinus
  » fistulae
  » warts
  » blood
  » discharge
    – colour
    – consistency
- Palpation
  » superficial and deep inguinal lymph nodes.

Cusco's speculum

▶ Inspect vagina and cervix for
  » erythema
  » ulceration
  » blood
  » discharge
    – colour
    – consistency
▶ Undertake high vaginal and two endocervical swabs (one for chlamydia).

Bimanual palpation

▶ Place one hand on lower abdomen to palpate
▶ With other hand, insert lubricated index and middle finger into the vagina
▶ Palpation
  » anterior and posterior fornices and adnexae
    – masses
    – cervical and adnexal tenderness
▶ Withdraw fingers and provide patient with tissue.

Additional bedside examinations and tests

▶ Review vital signs observation chart
▶ Urinalysis
▶ Fundoscopy
▶ Abdominal examination.

NOTES

CHAPTER 12

GYNAECOLOGY

In addition to using the general history, consider the following.

Incontinence

⮕ Does it occur when you . . .
- cough
- sneeze
- laugh?

⮕ Do you get an urge to pass water before you do pass water?

⮕ Do you have any warning before you pass water?

⮕ Does anything trigger the urge to go (i.e. putting the key into the front door)?

⮕ Does it stop you from doing things or going out?

⮕ Do you ever lose control of your bowels?

⮕ Do you have any numbness around your back passage?

⮕ Have you noticed any other changes when passing water, such as . . .
- burning or stinging sensation
- needing to pass water more often
- needing to pass water in the night?

Infertility

⮕ How long have you been trying to conceive?

- ➲ Do you or your partner have any children already?
- ➲ Are you having regular sex (at least twice a week)?
- ➲ How old were you when you had your first period?
- ➲ Do you currently have menstrual periods?
  - How many days between the first day of one period and the first day of the next?
  - If irregular: what is the shortest and longest length of periods?
- ➲ Have you been on any contraception in the past (i.e. depot injection)?
- ➲ Do you have excessive amount of hair in areas you would not expect (i.e. face, chest)?
- ➲ Have you ever had any discharge or milk from your nipples?
- ➲ Have you noticed any unintentional weight change?
- ➲ Do you experience any lower abdominal pain?
- ➲ Have you ever had a sexually transmitted disease?
- ➲ Have you ever had an ectopic pregnancy?
- ➲ Are there any emotional difficulties within the relationship?
- ➲ Does your partner have any illnesses/infections/take any medications/have a history of working with chemicals?
- ➲ Do either of you smoke?

Menstrual problems

- ➲ How many days between the first day of one period, and the first day of the next?
  - If irregular: what is the shortest and longest length of periods?
- ➲ What was the date of your last period?
- ➲ When did your periods start?
- ➲ How often do you have to change your sanitary towels/tampons a day?
  - Has this increased? When?
- ➲ Do you bleed between periods?

➲ Do you bleed after sex?

➲ Is sex painful?

➲ Have you had any accidents?

➲ Are there any blood clots?

➲ Is there any associated pain?

➲ Do you bleed from other areas (i.e. back passage) during your period?

➲ When was your last smear test?

➲ Have you had an abnormal smear in the past?

➲ Do you have any thyroid problems?

➲ Do you feel tired?

➲ Do you experience shortness of breath or chest pain?

➲ Is it stopping you from doing anything/going out?

➲ Do you use any form of contraception? Which (i.e. coil, depot)?

Pelvic pain

➲ How long have you had this pain?

➲ Does it coincide with your periods? If so, does it . . .

- start before your periods
- get worse or better when bleeding starts
- go when the bleeding stops?

➲ Do you have associated . . .

- heavy periods
- bleeding/spotting
- fever and feeling generally unwell
- change in bowel habits?

➲ Is there any possibility you may be pregnant?

➲ Do you have the coil fitted?

➲ Have you ever had unprotected sex?

➲ Have you had a sexually transmitted infection?

➲ Have you had any pelvic surgery?

➲ Have you had any change in bowel habit or in passing water?

Post-menopausal bleeding

➲ What bleeding have you had? For how long?

➲ How much are you bleeding?

- How many sanitary towels/tampons a day?

➲ Is it painful? Where?

➲ Is it only present when you pass water?

➲ Do you have a dragging sensation below?

➲ Have you unintentionally lost weight recently?

➲ When was your last smear? What was the result?

➲ Have you ever had an abnormal smear?

➲ Are you on/have you ever taken hormone replacement therapy?

➲ Have you ever had tamoxifen/had breast cancer?

➲ Did you have bleeding problems before the menopause?

➲ Have you ever had fertility problems?

Prolapse

➲ Do you have a dragging sensation below?

➲ Do you have back pain?

➲ Are you still having menstrual periods?

- Do you bleed between periods?

➲ Are you sexually active?

- Do you bleed after sex?

- Is sex painful?

➲ Have you had a period since menopause?

➲ Do you have any associated incontinence?

Vaginal discharge

➲ What colour is the discharge?

➲ Is it thin and watery or thick?

➲ Does it smell offensive (i.e. fishy)?

➲ Is there any associated . . .
- pain or irritation of the surrounding area
- pain on intercourse
- skin lesions?

➲ Have you been on any antibiotics recently?

➲ Do you have diabetes?

➲ Do you have any allergies?

➲ Has anything preceded it (i.e. sex, change of washing powder/ soap)?

➲ Have you recently changed sexual partners?

➲ How many sexual partners have you had over the past 12 months?

➲ Have you ever had unprotected sex?

Risk factors

Cervical cancer

➲ When was your last smear?

➲ Have you ever had an abnormal smear?

➲ Have you ever had unprotected sex?

➲ Have you ever been diagnosed with a sexually transmitted disease?

Ectopic pregnancy

➲ Do you have the coil fitted?

➲ Have you ever had . . .
- a sexually transmitted infection (i.e. chlamydia, gonorrhoea)
- pelvic surgery?

➲ Do you have endometriosis?

Endometrial cancer

➲ When was your first period?

➲ When was your last period?

- Do you have any children? How many?
- Did you breast feed?
- Are you taking hormone replacement therapy (oestrogen-only preparation)?
- Have you been treated for breast cancer with tamoxifen?
- Is there anyone in your family with breast, ovarian or womb cancer?
- Do you know what your weight is?
- Do you have . . .
  - diabetes
  - liver disease
  - hereditary non-polyposis colorectal carcinoma (HNPCC)/Lynch syndrome?

Incontinence/prolapse

- Do you have any children?
  - How many?
  - Did you have a prolonged/difficult labour?
  - Did you suffer any tearing from the labour?
- Do you have a . . .
  - connective tissue disorder
  - chronic cough?
- Do you know what your weight is?

GYNAECOLOGY EXAMINATION

General
- Introduction (name, grade)
- Explain examination
- Verbal consent
- Chaperone
- Wash hands/alcohol gel
- Wear gloves
- Patient to be lying and adequately exposed.

General bedside inspection
- Body habitus
- Patient discomfort or pain.

Groin
- Inspection
  - » erythema
  - » ulceration
  - » warts
  - » blood
  - » discharge
    - – colour
    - – consistency
- Palpation
  - » superficial and deep inguinal lymph nodes.

Cusco's speculum
- Inspect vagina and cervix for
  - » erythema
  - » ulceration

» blood
» discharge
  – colour
  – consistency
▶ Undertake high vaginal and two endocervical swabs (one for chlamydia).

If prolapse, Sim's speculum
▶ Patient in left lateral position, insert speculum along posterior vaginal wall
▶ Assess anterior and vault prolapse
▶ Slowly withdraw speculum and assess posterior vaginal wall prolapse.

Bimanual palpation
▶ Place one hand on lower abdomen to palpate
▶ With other hand, insert lubricated index and middle finger into the vagina
▶ Palpation
  » note uterine size and orientation
    – tenderness
  » lateral fornices and adnexae
    – masses
    – adnexal tenderness
    – cervical excitation pain
▶ Withdraw fingers and provide patient with tissue.

Additional bedside examinations and tests
▶ Review vital signs observation chart
▶ Breast examination[10]
▶ Abdominal examination.

CHAPTER 13

MUSCULOSKELETAL

In addition to using the general history, consider the following.

Instability

- ⮕ For how long has your affected area been unstable?
- ⮕ Did this follow an injury?
- ⮕ Which joint(s) are affected?
- ⮕ Has the instability caused you to fall?
- ⮕ Do you have/ever had . . .
  - a collagen disorder
  - sciatica/slipped disc
  - poliomyelitis?
- ⮕ Is there anyone in your family with joint instability?
- ⮕ Do you play any sports? Which?

Pain

- ⮕ When do you get your pain?
- ⮕ Where exactly is the pain?
- ⮕ How quickly did the pain start (suddenly or gradually)?
- ⮕ When is it most painful?
  - A particular movement or with all movements?
- ⮕ Does the pain change during the course of the day?
- ⮕ Does the pain wake you from sleep?

- ⊃ Does the pain get better or worse with movement?
- ⊃ Does it get better or worse with rest?
- ⊃ Is it associated with . . .
  - tingling or numbness
  - swelling
  - stiffness
  - shooting pain
  - loss of sensation
  - weakness?
- ⊃ Have you ever injured the affected area? When? How?
- ⊃ What does it stop you from doing?

Back

- ⊃ Is the pain in one area or widespread?
- ⊃ Is the pain constant or related to movement?
- ⊃ Does it get worse with bending forwards or backwards?
- ⊃ Is it associated with . . .
  - difficulty breathing
  - joint swelling
  - night pain
  - stiffness
  - skin rash
  - pain when passing water or passing water more frequently
  - pain anywhere in your abdomen?
- ⊃ Do you have . . .
  - cancer/myeloma
  - inflammatory bowel disease
  - cough and fever?
- ⊃ Have you ever lost control of your bladder or bowels?
- ⊃ Do you have any difficulty passing water?

⮞ When wiping yourself, does your back passage feel numb?

⮞ Have you unintentionally lost weight?

Limbs/hip

⮞ Is the pain on one side or both?

⮞ How many joints are affected?

⮞ Does it hurt to walk, stand, sit or lie?

Reduced movement

⮞ Is it pain that reduces movement of your affected area?

⮞ Are you limited to specific movements? All movements?

⮞ Does your affected area feel stuck?

⮞ Does your affected area dislocate?

Stiffness

⮞ Where does the stiffness affect you?

⮞ When are you most stiff?

⮞ How long does the stiffness last?

⮞ Does it restrict your movement?

⮞ Does it restrict your daily activities?

⮞ Does it improve with exercise?

⮞ Is there any associated pain in the affected area?

⮞ What job do you do/did you do?

⮞ Have you ever injured the affected area?

⮞ Have you noticed any rashes?

Back

⮞ Do you have any difficulties getting out of bed?

⮞ Is there any associated . . .

- rash
- heel pain/swelling

- eye problems (i.e. uveitis)
- breathing difficulty
- changes in bowel habit?

Swelling

⮑ How quickly did the swelling start (sudden or gradually)?

⮑ Where is the swelling?

⮑ How many joints are swollen?

⮑ Do the swollen areas look the same on both sides of your body?

⮑ Has the swelling been constant? Episodic?

⮑ Have you been using your [affected area] more repetitively recently?

⮑ Is the swelling associated with . . .
- stiffness
- pain
- white deposits of the joint
- feeling generally unwell
- lower back pain
- eye problems
- problems passing water
- fever/chills?

⮑ Have you injured the affected area?

Weakness

⮑ Where are you feeling weak?

⮑ Does the weakness fluctuate?

⮑ Does anything make it get worse/go away?

⮑ Does it restrict your daily activities?

⮑ Is there any associated loss of sensation?

⮑ Have you injured the affected area?

⮑ Is there anyone in your family with muscle disease?

➲ Are you taking medication such as . . .

- statins
- steroids?

Legs

➲ Do you have back pain?

➲ Have you ever lost control of your bladder?

➲ Have you ever lost control of your bowels?

➲ When you wipe yourself after using the toilet does your passage feel numb?

➲ Do you have cancer?

Risk factors

Carpal tunnel syndrome

➲ Which hand is affected? Is the other side affected?

➲ Which is your dominant hand?

➲ Have you ever injured your wrist?

➲ Do you have . . .

- inflammatory arthritis
- acromegaly
- diabetes
- underactive thyroid?

➲ Female: Are you pregnant?

➲ What is/was your occupation/hobbies? Are these affected?

Gout

➲ Do you drink alcohol? How much and for how long?

➲ What food would you eat on a typical day?

➲ Do you take any diuretics or water tablets?

➲ Do you have . . .

- kidney problems/failure
- leukaemia, myeloma or myelodysplastic syndrome?

Osteoarthritis

➲ How old are you?

➲ Have you ever injured the affected area?

➲ What job do you do/did you do in the past?

➲ Have you ever been overweight?

➲ Have you ever had . . .

- joint abnormalities from childhood
- inflammatory joint disease?

➲ Does arthritis run in your family?

Osteoporosis

➲ How old are you? When did you go through the menopause?

➲ Does osteoporosis run in your family?

➲ Do you smoke? How many and for how long?

➲ Do you drink alcohol? How much and for how long?

➲ Do you have any children?

➲ Are you, or were you, taking any long-term medication (steroids)?

➲ Do you have rheumatoid arthritis?

BACK EXAMINATION

General

- Introduction (name, grade)
- Explain examination
- Verbal consent
- Chaperone as appropriate
- Wash hands/alcohol gel
- Patient to be standing, then lying, and adequately exposed.

General bedside inspection

- Walking aids
- Discomfort/pain.

Inspection

- Anteriorly, posteriorly and laterally
  - » neck position (chin poke)
  - » scapular position
  - » rib hump
  - » symmetry of shoulders and pelvis
  - » leg position
  - » muscle atrophy/tone
  - » spina bifida
  - » axillary freckling
  - » exaggerated kyphosis and lordosis
  - » 'question mark' posture
  - » scoliosis
  - » scars
- Gait
  - » ataxia, antalgia, high steppage and swing out
    - – walking on tiptoes (S1)

- walking on heels (L5)
- squatting and standing (L3–5, S1)
- walking heel to toe (ataxia).

Palpation

▶ Temperature changes
▶ Tenderness
  » occiput to sacrum, along spinous processes and paravertebral muscles
  » palpate for sacroiliac and iliolumbar region tenderness
▶ Chest expansion.

Movement

▶ Neck movements
  » flexion/extension
  » looking right and left
  » movement of head towards shoulders
▶ Lumbar spine movements
  » flexion (Schober's test[11])
  » extension
  » lateral flexion
  » fix pelvis (or ask patient to sit) and rotate torso either side
▶ Leg movements (patient lying)
  » passive straight leg raise
    - dorsiflex ankle in straight leg raise (Lasègue's test)
    - pressure in popliteal fossa (bow string)
  » flex knee in straight leg raise to relieve pain.

Additional bedside examinations and tests

▶ Review vital signs observation chart
▶ Upper and lower limb neurovascular examinations.

SHOULDER EXAMINATION

General
▶ Introduction (name, grade)
▶ Explain examination
▶ Verbal consent
▶ Chaperone as appropriate
▶ Wash hands/alcohol gel
▶ Patient to be standing and adequately exposed.

General bedside inspection
▶ Patient discomfort/pain.

Inspection
▶ Anteriorly, posteriorly and laterally
  » posture (including scapulae position)
  » muscle wasting
  » skin changes
  » asymmetry
  » swelling.

Palpation
▶ Anteriorly and posteriorly
  » temperature changes
  » position of the humeral head
  » bony tenderness
    – anteriorly: sternoclavicular joint > clavicle > acromioclavicular joint > acromion > coracoid process > scapula; joint line > humeral head
    – posteriorly: spine of scapula > lateral border > inferior aspect > medial border > superior aspect

- » muscle bulk:
  - – supraspinatus
  - – infraspinatus
  - – deltoid.

Movement

- ▶ Active and passive (note resistance and crepitus)
  - » flexion and extension
  - » abduction and adduction
    - – painful arc
  - » circumflexion
  - » internal and external rotation
- ▶ Rotator cuff muscles
  - » empty can test[12] (supraspinatus)
  - » external rotation against resistance (infraspinatus and teres minor)
  - » belly press test[13] (subscapularis).

Additional bedside examinations and tests

- ▶ Hawkin's test[14]
- ▶ Scarf test[15]
- ▶ Upper limb neurovascular examination
- ▶ Cervical spine examination
- ▶ Elbow examination.

ELBOW EXAMINATION

General

▶ Introduction (name, grade)
▶ Explain examination
▶ Verbal consent
▶ Chaperone as appropriate
▶ Wash hands/alcohol gel
▶ Patient to be sitting and adequately exposed.

General bedside inspection

▶ Patient discomfort/pain.

Inspection

▶ Posture
  » carrying angle
  » fixed flexion deformity
▶ Swellings
  » rheumatic nodules
  » gouty tophi
  » bursitis
▶ Skin changes
  » psoriatic plaques
  » scars
▶ Symmetry.

Palpation

▶ Temperature changes
▶ Bony tenderness (lateral and medial epicondyles; olecranon process; radial head)
▶ Joint line tenderness

- Nodules
- Boggy swelling.

Movement

- Active and passive (note resistance and crepitus)
  - » flexion and extension
  - » supination and pronation
  - » internal and external rotation
- Assess for tennis elbow[16]
- Assess for golfer's elbow.[17]

Additional bedside examinations and tests

- Shoulder examination
- Hand/wrist examination
- Upper limb neurovascular examination.

HAND AND WRIST EXAMINATION

General
- Introduction (name, grade)
- Explain examination
- Verbal consent
- Chaperone as appropriate
- Wash hands/alcohol gel
- Patient to be sitting and adequately exposed.

General bedside inspection
- Patient discomfort/pain

Inspection
- Erythema
- Nail pitting/onycholysis
- Psoriatic plaques
- A/symmetrical dactylitis
- Deformities
  - » ulnar deviation
  - » fixed flexion deformity of fingers
  - » swan neck deformity
  - » Boutonniere deformity
  - » Z-shaped deformity
  - » Heberden's (DIPJ) and Bouchard's (PIPJ) nodes
  - » subluxation at carpo-metacarpophalangeal joints.

Palpation
- Temperature changes
- Tenderness, swelling or instability
  - » distal interphalangeal joints (DIPJ)

- » proximal interphalangeal joints (PIPJ)
- » metacarpophalangeal joints
- » carpo-metacarpal joints
- » carpo-metacarpophalangeal joints
- » carpal bones
- ▶ Boggy swelling over dorsum of hand
- ▶ Sensation
  - » radial nerve distribution (1st web space on dorsum of hand)
  - » median nerve distribution (radial border of index finger)
  - » ulnar nerve distribution (ulnar border of little finger).

Movement

- ▶ Radial nerve distribution
  - » wrist extension (extensor carpi radialis (longus and brevis), extensor carpi ulnaris and extensor digitorum)
  - » finger extension (extensor digitorum, extensor indicis and extensor digiti minimi)
  - » thumb extension (extensor pollicis longus and brevis)
- ▶ Median nerve distribution
  - » resist thumb abduction (abductor pollicis brevis)
- ▶ Ulnar nerve distribution
  - » abduction and adduction of fingers (dorsal and palmar interossei)
  - » little finger abduction (abductor digiti minimi)
  - » Froment's sign[18] (adductor pollicis)
- ▶ Range of movement of wrist
- ▶ Hand function
  - » grip strength
  - » key grip
  - » opposition strength
  - » practical ability.

Additional bedside examinations and tests

- Special tests for carpal tunnel:
  - » Tinel's test[19]
  - » Phalen's test[20]
- Elbow examination
- Upper limb neurovascular examination.

HIP EXAMINATION

General

▶ Introduction (name, grade)

▶ Explain examination

▶ Verbal consent

▶ Chaperone as appropriate

▶ Wash hands/alcohol gel

▶ Patient to be standing, then lying and adequately exposed.

General bedside inspection

▶ Walking aids

▶ Discomfort/pain.

Inspection

▶ Gait

  » ataxia

  » antalgia

  » high steppage

  » swing out

▶ Leg position on standing

▶ Asymmetry

▶ Muscle wasting

▶ Bony deformity

▶ Swelling

▶ Rotation

▶ True and apparent limb lengths

▶ Trendelenburg's test.[21]

Palpation

▶ Temperature changes

- Bony tenderness (greater trochanter and femur shaft)
- Joint line tenderness
- Muscle bulk
- Thomas test[22] for fixed flexion deformity.

Movement

- Active and passive movement (note crepitus)
  - » flexion and extension
  - » abduction and adduction
  - » internal and external rotation.

Additional bedside examinations and tests

- Spine examination
- Knee examination
- Lower limb neurovascular examination.

KNEE EXAMINATION

General

▶ Introduction (name, grade)

▶ Explain examination

▶ Verbal consent

▶ Chaperone as appropriate

▶ Wash hands/alcohol gel

▶ Patient to be standing, then lying, and adequately exposed.

General bedside inspection

▶ Walking aids

▶ Discomfort/pain.

Inspection

▶ Standing posture

▶ Valgus/varus deformity

▶ Fixed flexion/hyperextension deformity

▶ Squatting posture

▶ Swelling

▶ Muscle atrophy

▶ Skin changes

▶ Gait

» ataxia

» antalgia

» high steppage

» swing out.

Palpation

▶ Temperature changes

▶ Patella tap/ballot

- Joint line tenderness
- Bony tenderness (femoral condyles; patella; patella tendon; tibial tuberosity)
- Hamstrings.

Movement

- Active and passive movement (note restriction and crepitus)
  - » flexion and extension
- Ligament stability
  - » lateral and medial collateral ligaments
  - » Anterior and posterior drawer tests.[23]

Additional bedside examinations and tests

- McMurray's special test[24]
- Hip examination
- Ankle examination
- Lower limb neurovascular examination.

FOOT/ANKLE EXAMINATION

General

- Introduction (name, grade)
- Explain examination
- Verbal consent
- Chaperone as appropriate
- Wash hands/alcohol gel
- Patient to be lying and adequately exposed.

General bedside inspection

- Inspect shoes for uneven wear and insoles
- Walking aids
- Discomfort/pain.

Inspection

- Toes
  - » valgus deformity
  - » varus deformity
  - » clawing
  - » hammer toes
- Foot arches
  - » pes planus/planovalgus
    - – 'too many toes' sign
    - – correctable on tiptoe
  - » pes cavus/cavovarus
- Nails
  - » pitting
  - » onycholysis
- Swellings
  - » callus

- » gouty tophi
- » rheumatic nodules
- » ganglion
- » synovitis
- » retrocalcaneal bursitis
- » enthesitis
- ▶ Skin changes
- ▶ Gait.

Palpation

- ▶ Temperature change
- ▶ Achilles tendon
  - » tenderness
  - » thickening
  - » insertion/gap
- ▶ Bony tenderness
  - » metatarsophalangeal joints
  - » subtalar joint
  - » malleolar zone
    - – distal 6 cm of the posterior edge of the tibia or tip of the medial malleolus
    - – distal 6 cm of the posterior edge of the fibula or tip of the lateral malleolus
  - » midfoot zone
    - – base of the fifth metatarsal
    - – navicular bone
- ▶ Peripheral pulses
  - » dorsalis pedis
  - » posterior tibialis.

Movement

- Active and passive movement (note resistance and crepitus)
  - » dorsiflexion and plantarflexion
    - – ankle
    - – toes
  - » inversion and eversion
    - – midfoot
    - – forefoot.

Additional bedside examinations and tests

- Simmonds–Thompson test[25]
- Knee examination
- Lower limb neurovascular examination.

CHAPTER 14

SKIN, NAILS AND HAIR

In addition to using the general history, consider the following.

Hair loss

- ➲ Was the hair loss sudden or gradual?
- ➲ Does the loss occur only on the scalp or is the body hair involved as well?
- ➲ Is the baldness localised or general, symmetrical or asymmetrical?
- ➲ Is there a family history of baldness (especially in men)?
- ➲ What drugs have you taken recently?
- ➲ Any recent illness, stress or trauma?
- ➲ Female: Have you recently had a baby?
- ➲ Are there other symptoms (hypothyroidism, acne, abnormal menses)?

Hirsutism

- ➲ Does anyone in your family have excessive hair growth?
- ➲ Are your menstrual periods normal and regular?
- ➲ Do you experience visual disturbances or headaches?
- ➲ Do you take medications (phenytoin, anabolic steroids, progestogens)?

Skin lesion(s)

- ➲ How quickly did the lesion develop (suddenly or gradually)?
- ➲ Is the skin itchy or painful?
- ➲ Has it changed in size or shape since you first noticed it?
- ➲ Is there any associated discharge (blood or pus)?
- ➲ Have you recently taken any antibiotics or other drugs?
- ➲ Have you used any creams or topical medications?
- ➲ Were there any preceding symptoms such as fever, sore throat, anorexia, vaginal discharge?
- ➲ Have you travelled abroad recently? Were you bitten by insects?
- ➲ Any possible exposure to industrial or domestic skin irritants or allergens?
- ➲ Any possible contact with sexually transmitted disease or HIV?
- ➲ Have you had close physical contact with others with skin disorders?

Risk factors

Basal cell and squamous cell carcinoma

- ➲ Have you had excessive sun exposure?
- ➲ What is/was your occupation?
- ➲ Were you ever sunburnt as a child?
- ➲ Have you ever had skin cancer?
- ➲ Do you have . . .
  - cancer
  - diabetes
  - HIV
  - actinic keratosis
  - skin ulcers?

Eczema

⮕ Do you have . . .

- asthma
- hay fever
- allergies?

⮕ Does anyone in your family have . . .

- eczema
- asthma
- hay fever
- allergies?

⮕ Do you work . . .

- with chemicals
- with biological hazards
- with animals
- in excessive heat or cold?

Malignant melanoma

⮕ Is this a new mole or an old one that has changed shape/size?

⮕ Have you ever had a melanoma?

⮕ Do you have psoriasis? Do you take oral psoralens or PUVA for it?

⮕ Do you have . . .?

- cancer
- diabetes
- HIV?

⮕ Have you had excessive sun exposure?

⮕ Have you burnt in the sun in the past?

⮕ Has anyone in your family had a melanoma?

LUMPS/BUMPS EXAMINATION

General

▶ Introduction (name, grade)

▶ Explain examination

▶ Verbal consent

▶ Chaperone as appropriate

▶ Wash hands/alcohol gel

▶ Patient to be sitting or lying and adequately exposed.

General bedside inspection

▶ Overlying skin

  » erythematous

  » bruised

  » sinuses/fistulae

  » lacerations/abrasions.

Inspection

▶ Number, distribution and configuration

▶ Describe:

  » site

  » size

  » tenderness

  » shape

  » surface (e.g. smooth/lumpy)

  » edges (e.g. smooth/hard/nodular/well circumscribed)

  » scars

  » discharge

▶ *Pigmented lesions*

  » asymmetry

  » border irregularity

» >2 colours
» diameter >7 mm.

Palpation

▶ Tenderness
▶ Temperature
▶ Consistency (e.g. soft/firm/hard/irregular)
▶ Fluctuance
▶ Pulsatility
▶ Compressibility
▶ Reducibility
▶ Fixity (to deep structures, e.g. underlying muscles)
▶ Tethering (to skin).

Additional bedside examinations and tests

▶ Transilluminate or auscultate for bruits, if appropriate
▶ Examine local lymph nodes
▶ Examine distal neurovascular supply.

ULCER EXAMINATION

General
▶ Introduction (name, grade)
▶ Explain examination
▶ Verbal consent
▶ Chaperone as appropriate
▶ Wash hands/alcohol gel
▶ Patient to be sitting or lying and adequately exposed.

General bedside inspection
▶ Overlying skin
    » erythema
    » cellulitis.

Inspection
▶ Site
▶ Size
▶ Tenderness
▶ Shape
▶ Depth
▶ Edges
    » sloping
    » punched out
    » undermined
    » rolled
    » everted
▶ Base
    » healthy
    » sloughy
    » avascular

» purulent

» necrotic

» underlying structures visible.

Additional bedside examinations and tests

▶ Examine regional lymph nodes

▶ Vascular examination, as appropriate

▶ Neurological examination.

NOTES

CHAPTER 15

PSYCHIATRY

Affective and neurotic symptoms

Mood

- How would you describe your mood?
- Do you feel worse at any particular time of day?
- Do you have difficulty getting off to sleep?
- Do you wake up early in the morning?
- How is your appetite?
- What do you enjoy doing?
- Have you lost interest in any of your usual activities?
- Has your energy level changed recently?
- Do you find it difficult to concentrate?
- Have you lost interest in love making?
- How does the future seem to you?

Mania

- How much have you slept recently?
- Do you find it difficult to keep still for any length of time?
- Have you started any new projects or activities recently?
- Have you been spending more money than usual?

Anxiety

⮞ Do you ever feel anxious for no particular reason?

⮞ Do you sometimes feel tense or 'on edge'?

⮞ Do you find yourself worrying about trivial matters?

⮞ Do you ever have the feeling that you, or the world about you, is unreal?

⮞ Do you ever get sudden feelings of panic?

⮞ Does anything trigger these feelings?

⮞ Are there times when you . . .

- feel shaky
- sweat a lot
- feel that you are choking
- feel that your heart is pounding
- get a churning sensation in your stomach?

⮞ Do these feelings stop you from doing things?

Obsessional thoughts and compulsive acts

⮞ Do unwelcome thoughts keep entering your mind even though you struggle against them?

⮞ Do you have to repeat any actions many times and in exactly the same order?

Self-harm

⮞ Do you feel that life is worth living?

⮞ Have you ever thought of ending your life?

⮞ What ways of hurting or killing yourself have you thought of?

⮞ Does anything trigger these thoughts?

⮞ What has prevented you from committing suicide?

Psychotic symptoms

It is useful to first introduce the questions about psychotic symptoms, such as: 'I would like to ask you some questions that we ask everyone

who comes to us. Some of the questions may appear a bit strange.
Please tell me if you are not sure what they mean.'

Hallucinations

⮥ Do you ever hear things that other people cannot hear and no
   ordinary explanation seems possible?
⮥ Do you ever hear voices when there is nobody about?
   ● How many voices are there?
   ● Do you recognise them?
   ● Do they talk to you or about you?
   ● Do the voices give you instructions?
   ● Do you feel that you must obey them?
⮥ Do you ever see things that other people cannot see or experience
   bodily sensations that you cannot account for?

Delusions

⮥ Do you have the feeling that something odd is going on but you
   are not sure what it is?
⮥ Is any person, or group of people, trying to harm you or make your
   life miserable?
⮥ Do you feel forced to defend yourself?
⮥ Do you think that someone is spying on you or following you?
⮥ Is there any reference to you in the newspaper or on radio or
   television?
⮥ Do you feel that you have any special talents or powers that
   ordinary people lack?

Passivity experiences

⮥ Do you think that your thoughts or actions are controlled by an
   outside agency?
⮥ Is there something like X-rays or radio waves affecting your body?

➲ Do you sometimes feel like a puppet or robot controlled by someone and without a will of your own?

Past psychiatric history

➲ Have you ever been treated by your general practitioner for a mental illness such as anxiety or depression?
➲ Were you prescribed medication? If so, can you remember the name of it? Did your GP refer you for talking therapy with either a counsellor or a psychotherapist?
➲ Have you ever tried to harm yourself, for example, by taking an overdose?
➲ Have you ever been in contact with the psychiatric services?
➲ Have you ever been admitted to a psychiatric ward? Do you know if this was under the Mental Health Act?

Personal history

Infancy, childhood and adolescence

➲ Where were you born?
➲ Were there any problems associated with your birth?
➲ Did you learn to walk and talk at the normal ages?
➲ Were you ever separated from your parents?
➲ What is your favourite childhood memory?
➲ What is your worst childhood memory?
➲ How did you get on with your mum and dad?
➲ Did you have any major problems as a teenager?

If a history of abuse is suspected further questioning is required:

'I am going to ask you about some unpleasant things that happen to some people in childhood. We ask because sometimes it throws light on difficulties later in life. It's fine if you prefer not to answer these questions.'

- ⮡ When you were a child, did anyone hurt or punish you in a way that left bruises, cuts or scratches?
- ⮡ When you were a child, did anyone ever do something sexual that made you feel uncomfortable?

Education
- ⮡ How old were you when you started school?
- ⮡ What types of school did you attend?
- ⮡ Did you have any specific difficulties at school, e.g. in reading or arithmetic?
- ⮡ Did you have any friends at school?
- ⮡ Were you bullied or teased much?
- ⮡ How did you get on with the teachers?
- ⮡ Did you ever play truant?
- ⮡ Were you ever suspended or expelled from school?
- ⮡ What qualifications did you get?

Occupational record
- ⮡ Starting from when you left school, what jobs have you had since?
- ⮡ How long did you work for in each job?
- ⮡ Why did you change jobs?
- ⮡ Did you get along with your colleagues in each job? What did you think of them?
- ⮡ Did you get along with your boss in each job? What did you think of them?

Psychosexual development and relationships
- ⮡ When was your first sexual experience?
- ⮡ Have you had any unpleasant sexual experiences?
- ⮡ Have you ever had a same-sex relationship?
- ⮡ Does sex or your own sexuality cause you any anxieties?

⮕ Are you currently in a relationship? How would you describe it?

⮕ How would you describe your previous relationships? Why do you think they did not last?

⮕ Do you have any children? How do you interact with them?

Alcohol/illicit drugs

⮕ Do you like drinking alcohol?

⮕ How old were you when you started drinking?

⮕ Have your drinking habits changed?

⮕ Has alcohol caused any major problems in your life?

⮕ Have you ever experimented with illicit drugs such as cannabis, amphetamine, ecstasy, LSD, cocaine or heroin?

- How old were you when you first took drugs?

- Some people take drugs to escape from their problems or to fit in with the people around them. What do you think led you to take drugs?

Forensic

⮕ Have you ever been in trouble with the police? If so, for what?

⮕ Have you any previous convictions?

⮕ Have you ever been on probation or served a prison sentence? If so, what for?

⮕ Have you any court case pending?

Present circumstances

⮕ What sort of accommodation do you have at the moment? Are there any problems with it?

⮕ Who do you live with? Are you on good terms with them?

⮕ Are you working at the moment? How do you find your job?

⮕ Do you have any financial problems?

⮕ Do you have many friends?

- Do you partake in any leisure activities?
- On average, how much alcohol do you drink per week?
- Are you currently taking any illicit drugs?
- Describe a typical day in your life.

Family history

- Have any of your relatives suffered from a mental illness such as depression, schizophrenia or dementia?
- Have any of your relatives suffered from an alcohol or drug problem?
- Have any members of your family tried to harm themselves?

Premorbid personality

- In the past how have other people described you? How would you describe yourself?
- In what ways are you like your mother and father? In what ways are you different from them?
- Do you have any guiding philosophy in life?
- Do you have a faith? How important is this faith to you?

MENTAL STATE EXAMINATION

If not already covered in the history.

General
- Introduction (name, grade)
- Explain examination
- Verbal consent.

General bedside inspection
- Psychomotor retardation/agitation
- Repetitive movements
- Absent facies.

Appearance and behaviour
- Well-kempt/unkempt
- Psychomotor retardation/agitation
- Maintains/avoids eye contact
- Involuntary movements.

Speech
- Rate, rhythm, tone and content
- Thought disorder (e.g. pressure of speech, derailment, tangentiality, illogicality).

Affect/mood
- Range of affect
- Obtain subjective interpretation of mood
- Provide objective interpretation of mood.

Thought

▶ Form and content
▶ Assess for thoughts of self-harm or harm to others (SAD PERSONS scale[26])

Perception

▶ Enquire about hallucinations, especially auditory and visual.

Cognition

▶ Assess if orientated to person, time and place
▶ Abbreviated mental test[27]/mini mental state examination if appropriate.

Insight

▶ Ask if the patient thinks that . . .
  » they are unwell
  » their experiences could be due to a mental illness
  » their condition could be improved with treatments such as psychotropic medication or psychotherapy?

NOTES

APPENDIX 1

SPECIFIC TESTS, SCALES AND EXAMINATIONS

1 Buerger's test

1 Patient lying; raise lower limb slowly, one at a time
2 Note at what angle the following is observed in the feet/legs:
   - blanching
   - guttering of veins
   - *up to 90 degrees is normal, <50 degrees severe ischaemia, <25 degrees critical ischaemia*
3 Lower the legs steadily and allow them to swing down to the floor (sitting the patient up as you go)
4 Observe the foot for a red/purple discolouration.

2 Trendelenburg's/tourniquet test

1 With patient lying flat, elevate one leg and milk blood from veins
2 Apply pressure at saphenofemoral junction (SFJ) with your fingers (Trendelenburg) or tourniquet
3 Ask patient to stand:
   - if varicosities are controlled, valvular incompetence is at SFJ

- if varicosities refill, valvular incompetence is distal to the SFJ:
  - repeat and apply pressure progressively distally until varicosities are controlled

3 Tap test

1 With patient standing, percuss SFJ and palpate for any transmitted percussions down the leg.

4 Digital rectal examination

Fully explain procedure and obtain consent. Chaperone must be present. Patient to be positioned in left lateral decubitus with hips and knees flexed. Wear gloves. Communicate to patient what you are doing at each stage.

1 Inspect anus for:
- inflammation
- skin tags
- excoriations
- fistulae
- fissures
- ulceration
- haemorrhoids

2 Lubricate finger and insert into rectum
- Palpate for:
  - masses
  - prostate abnormalities
- Assess sphincter tone

3 Remove finger and inspect glove for:
- faeces
- blood

- mucus
- melaena

4 Wipe the patient and leave them with additional tissue.

5 Hernial orifice examination

Patient to be lying first, then standing.

1 Inspect hernia and surrounding skin; note location:
- superior and medial to pubic tubercle (inguinal)
- inferior and lateral to pubic tubercle (femoral)
2 Palpate to assess if reducible or incarcerated –

  If reducible:
- inspect for cough impulse without pressure over reduced hernia
- inspect for cough impulse with pressure over reduced hernia
3 Ask patient to stand
- inspect for reappearance of hernia
4 For completion:
- abdominal examination
- contralateral groin examination.

6 Rinne's test

1 Apply the base of a vibrating 512 Hz tuning fork to mastoid process
2 Ask the patient to acknowledge when they can no longer hear the sound
3 Remove the tuning fork and place in front of auditory meatus
4 Ask patient if they can hear the sound
5 Repeat this test for both ears.

7 Weber's test

1 Apply the base of a vibrating 512 Hz tuning fork to the midline of the forehead

2 Ask the patient if they can hear the sound loudest in one ear over the other, or if the sound is equal.

8 Romberg's test

1 Ask patient to stand feet together and close their eyes.

9 Unterberger's test

1 Ask patient to hold arms out straight, march on the spot, and close their eyes.

10 Breast examination

Patient to be sitting first then lying. Chaperone must be present.

1 With patient sitting, inspect for:

  a Asymmetry of breasts

  b Skin changes – tethering, puckering, peau d'orange

  c Nipple discharge/bleeding

  d Obvious deformity (e.g. nipple inversion)

2 Repeat inspection with:

  a Patient's arms above her head

  b Patient's hands pushing into her waist

3 Ask patient to lie down with one hand positioned behind her head:

  a Palpate:

    i All four quadrants of breast

    ii Nipple

    iii Axillary lymph nodes

4 Repeat palpation on other breast, with patient's other hand behind her head

5 Cover patient with blanket

6 For completion
  - Palpation
    - hepatosplenomegaly
    - bony tenderness of spine
  - Respiratory examination.

11 Schober's test

1 With patient standing, mark L5 (level of posterior iliac spine)

2 Place one finger 5 cm below L5 and another finger 10 cm above L5

3 Ask patient to bend over to touch their toes.

12 Empty can test

1 Ask patient to bring arms out straight with thumbs pointing downwards

2 Arms should be approximately 45 degrees from the legs

3 Push down onto the patient's arms, instructing them to resist your pressure.

13 Belly press test

1 Ask patient to place both hands on their abdomen with their elbows pointing forwards

2 Push back onto the patient's elbows, instructing them to resist your pressure.

14 Hawkin's test

1 Abduct patient's arm to 90 degrees and flex elbow to 90 degrees
2 Flex shoulder to 30 degrees (with elbow still flexed)
3 Stabilise arm and internally rotate shoulder.

15 Scarf test

1 Flex patient's arm 90 degrees
2 Adduct patient's arm across the body.

16 Tennis elbow assessment

1 With elbow flexed, ask patient to extend wrist
2 Assess for tenderness or pain over lateral epicondyle.

17 Golfer's elbow assessment

1 With elbow flexed, ask patient to flex wrist
2 Assess for tenderness over medial epicondyle.

18 Froment's sign

1 Ask patient to keep hold of a piece of paper between their thumbs
   and fingers as you try to pull the paper away
2 Ask patient to keep their thumbs straight.

19 Tinel's test

1 Tap over carpal tunnel of affected hand.

20 Phalen's test

1 Ask patient to push dorsal surfaces of both hands together.

21 Trendelenburg's test

1 Place hands on patient's hips and ask patient to hold onto your arms

2 Ask patient to lift up one leg at a time.

22 Thomas test

1 With patient lying, put hand under patient's back

2 Ask patient to lift up one leg at a time.

23 Anterior and posterior drawer tests

1 Patient lying with knee flexed

2 Stabilise foot and pull/push tibia.

24 McMurray's test

1 Patient lying with hip and knee flexed 90 degrees

2 Extend and flex knee in both medial and lateral rotation.

25 Simmonds–Thompson test

1 Patient lying prone

2 Squeeze calf.

26 SAD PERSONS scale

Sex Male	1
Age <19 years or >45 years	1
Depression or hopelessness	2
Previous suicide attempts or psychiatric care	1
Excessive alcohol or drug use	1
Rational thinking loss (psychotic or organic illness)	2
Separated, widowed or divorced	1
Organised or serious attempt	2
No social support	1
Stated future attempt	2

27 Abbreviated mental test

I would like to ask you some questions to test your memory. You will probably find some questions easier to answer than others. Don't worry if you don't know the answer.

How old are you?	1
What is the time to the nearest hour?	1
Please remember the following address: 42 West Street	
What year is it?	1
What building are we in?	1
Can you identify the jobs of two people here?	1
What is your date of birth?	1
In what year did World War I begin?	1
Who is the present monarch?	1
Please count backwards from 20 to 1	1
Can you please tell me the address I asked you to remember?	1

Index

eyelid retraction 50
eyes, in acromegaly examination 45

face/neck
    in cardiovascular examination 13
    in diabetic examination 47
    in gastrointestinal examination 36
    in general examination 6–7
    in renal examination 63
    in respiratory examination 26
    in thyroid examination 50
face pain 79–80
facial appearance, changes in 39–40, 42
facial features, coarse 44
facial nerve 71, 89
facial weakness 66, 70, 79
facies, absent 152
family history 2, 73, 137, 151
farming industry 23
fasciculation 72, 74, 76
febrile convulsions 69
feet; *see also* legs/feet examination
    deformities in 47
    rest pain in 15
fever
    in gastrointestinal examination 31–2
    in general examination 3
    and infections 54
    and menstrual problems 109
    in renal examination 57–8
    in respiratory examination 21–2
    and skin lesions 138
    and swelling 118
fluorescein staining 94
foetor
    of ketosis 46
    uraemic 63
foetor hepaticus/oris 36
foot and ankle examination 134–6
foot arches 134
forehead bossing 44
forensic history 150
Froment's sign 128, 160
fundoscopy
    in cardiovascular examination 14
    and cranial nerves 70
    in diabetic examination 48
    in genitourinary inspection 101, 105
    in ophthalmological examination 95
    in renal examination 64
fungal infection 47

gag reflex 71
gait, inspection of 121–2, 130, 132
galactorrhoea 39–40
gastroenteritis 99
gastrointestinal examination 35–6
general examination 6–8
genitourinary examination
    female 102, 104
    male 97, 100–1
glaucoma 93
glomerulonephritis 59
glossitis 36, 55
glossopharyngeal nerve 71
glue-sniffing 84
goitre 7, 49–50
golfer's elbow 126, 160
gout 60, 119
gouty tophi 62, 125, 135
groin, inspection of 100, 113
GTN spray 9, 17, 19
gynaecology examination 113–14
gynaecomastia 36, 100

haematological examination 55–6
haematuria, visual 58
haemorrhoids 31, 156
haemosiderin staining 19
hair; *see also* body hair
    absence of 47
    dry 40, 42
hair loss 17, 137
hallucinations 147, 153
hammer toes 134
hand and wrist examination 126–9
hand function 128
hands, spade-like 44
hands/arms
    in acromegaly examination 44–5
    in cardiovascular examination 12
    in diabetic examination 46
    in gastrointestinal examination 35
    in general examination 6
    in renal examination 62
    in respiratory examination 25
    in thyroid examination 49
Hawkin's test 124, 160
hay fever 84, 139
head injury 41, 67–9